Advance Praise for *Trapped!*

"As a psychotherapist, I'm grateful to Nathan Joblin for writing *Trapped!*. This material is timely, given that some of our culture's voices can mischaracterize the masculine as solely toxic, leaving many feeling misunderstood and maligned. This book speaks to the need for compassion, courage, and strength in addressing the healing and health of the masculine. Nathan Joblin's work is a pathway forward for men looking to shift/free themselves toward a new paradigm of grounding their lives in purpose, meaning, and love. *Trapped!* is a must-read to awaken and support the heroic masculine, a crucial and valuable part of the human collective."

– **Natasha Senra-Pereira,** MSW, RSW, RP, Social Worker, Psychotherapist, Author/Speaker

"Many men will feel a deep resonance with Nathan Joblin and the feeling of being trapped in roles they have created for themselves. Rather than offering glib advice or a 'quick fix,' this book provides practical guidance to help us find deep satisfaction and purpose in our lives, creating fulfillment for ourselves as we support and nurture those we care about."

– **Bryan Welch,** author of *Beautiful and Abundant, Building the World We Want*
Co-CEO, Silk Grass Holdings US
Former CEO, Mindful Communications

"*Trapped!* is for men who feel stuck in their financial obligations and routines and want to find their way back to a sense of liberation. The book offers a direct and simple approach filled with practical tips, exercises, and strategies readers can use to break out and break free. Nathan Joblin emphasizes the importance of taking responsibility for one's own life and making conscious choices aligned with one's values and goals. He provides guidance on how to set boundaries, communicate effectively with others, and cultivate healthy habits supporting personal growth. I know many men who have fallen into the TRAP and highly recommend this book."

– **Paul Lemberg,** author of *Be Unreasonable*,
business mentor, and Entrepreneurial Shaman

"In an age where marriages and communities crumble, partially because we have not welcomed men in their wholeness, *Trapped!* is an essential exploration of healthy masculinity. It's evident when an author is committed to his reader's transformation. In *Trapped!*, Joblin is intentional with every word, which means there is no fluff. His material is relatable and informative, effortlessly leading to the practices that undoubtedly will set a trapped man free."

– **Alana Fournet,** best-selling author of *Radiant Powerful You*

"*Trapped!* offers practical, accessible steps men can take to grow into their fuller selves. Joblin's trustworthy guidance has the mark of a man who clearly knows this territory."

– **Reuvain Bacal,** MA, Transformational Men's Coach

"*Trapped!* is a must-read for the man who has achieved success yet feels empty and unfulfilled. It gives a simple-to-understand yet profound blueprint for finding meaning beyond career and family. Through cultivating awareness, accountability, and intentional action, Joblin gives us the tools to cultivate authentic and meaningful power and purpose in our lives."

– **Dent Gitchel,** PhD, LPC, author of *Pursuing Purpose*
Certified Teacher of *Compassion Cultivation Training &* Instructor
in *Mindfulness-Based Emotional Balance*

TRAPPED!

The Responsible Man's Guide to PERSONAL FREEDOM AND HAPPINESS

NATHAN JOBLIN

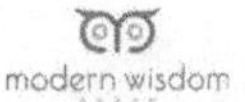

PRESS

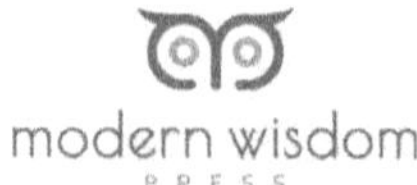

Modern Wisdom Press
Boulder, Colorado, USA
www.modernwisdompress.com

Cover design by Melinda Martin
Author's photo courtesy of Tracy VanDover

ISBN: 978-1-951692-32-2 (paperback), 978-1-951692-33-9 (epub)

For my children—Celie and Aiden—
for being patient with me
and inspiring me to be a better person.

For Catherine—
I wouldn't, and couldn't, do this without you.

CONTENTS

INTRODUCTION

This book is a hand outstretched to men who feel trapped. It's an invitation to those who've lost their way along the path they envisioned for their lives. Those hard workers who have checked off all the boxes but now find themselves constricted, even resentful, feeling the weight of responsibilities and the obligation to fulfill everyone's needs but their own.

Many of us earn the label of people pleaser. We are dependable employees. We show up when and where we are expected. We pick up the slack. We don't tend to connect too deeply with others, certainly not from a position of vulnerability. We have been taught to wear a mask of stoicism, no matter what we feel inside. Yet, through the last couple of decades and now into my fifties, I have found that I need authentic connections in my life to learn how to express myself fully, and so do other people in similar life stages and circumstances. Experiencing each day with realness and rawness was never part of our programming, yet I have discovered it is crucial to feeling alive.

American men who have some financial stability and do not have to spend each day battling class- or race-based oppression have immense personal power and potential control over their lives. Yet many of us experience ourselves as victims and blame our unhappiness and dissatisfaction on external situations and other people. We generally cannot accept the fact that we're wrong to search outside ourselves for the source of our unhappiness. I know I could not accept responsibility for my own well-being for a very long time.

I had no idea how to free myself from the constant effort of trying to get by. Then, just when I thought I would be stuck in the same unsatisfying, draining place forever, things began to shift. Slowly, by fits and starts, I learned how to address my demons and negative patterns and redirect the energy I had previously used to barely get by to engage in life in a way that inspired me to thrive. I hope that by writing down my experience of our common challenges, this book will encourage men feeling trapped by their external responsibilities to explore life in new ways—ways that will lead them to prioritize their responsibility to themselves.

Many of us have the sense that we are isolated even in our busy, crowded lives. We might also feel misunderstood by every other person or unheard by those closest to us. These themes may ring a bell for you: work, marriage, family, success, stress, setbacks, chores, some adventure, and many scheduled routines. The days quickly fill themselves with all the things we must do, and before we know it, we can find ourselves stuck in the ruts we've carved into our own lives. But by looking at the big picture of your life, you can step outside the narrow story you carry with you about who you are and where your life is headed.

This book calls out to all the self-avowed responsible guys who feel trapped: get to know yourself more deeply and recognize that you are part of a greater whole. We all share the basic human desires for happiness and freedom. I hope that in these pages, you'll find deeper meaning in the life you've created and learn it's perfectly possible to experience liberation from your struggles and feel less alone. When you put yourself at the top of your list of responsibilities, living a life of happiness and freedom is within your power.

I am excited to be here with you as you explore a more profound understanding of your potential and personal power.

CHAPTER 1

○○○— — —○○○

The Responsible Man's Dilemma

If you're one of us, you have likely worked hard to get where you are. Your years of full-time employment might have come right on the heels of years of education. If you're a family man, you manage or share the responsibility of running a home that requires daily blood, sweat, and tears. Whether or not you have a mortgage, you have likely taken on some form of debt to help address your basic needs. You have acquired much of what is needed in our complex and unyielding society.

Your sense of self is probably tied to providing for others and accomplishing tasks large and small. After all, this is how you seem to spend every bit of your time. The stream of demands on you only seems to grow, and so far, you have embraced your situation with both hands. Many of us people pleasers have determined that it's easier to focus on everyone else's happiness than our own. Somehow that becomes the path of least resistance.

Yet beneath the facade of serving everyone else's needs, you're dissatisfied and perhaps even resentful. Maybe you've walked this tightrope of obligation for years, and slowly and seemingly inevitably, you're losing your grasp. It can be terrifying. What you thought mattered is ceasing to have real meaning.

The Paradox

The paradox is that while you may be providing for your financial needs, and those around you may feel supported by your efforts, you do not feel fulfilled. In this scenario, it's frequently true that the more we accomplish, the less we feel connected to a sense of real meaning and purpose in our lives.

This is because we have been working to achieve the wrong goals. When we measure ourselves by how much we do, how much money we make, and what roles we are filling, we will ultimately feel a persistent emptiness, regardless of how much praise we receive. The loudest voice in our head tells us that if we figure out how to keep everyone happy, we will be loved, feel safe, and earn respect. We imagine that we will have solved our problems.

The reason for this mismatch between how much you do and how you feel is that the role you are playing is simply that: a role. We can think of ourselves as actors engaged in a performance or—on darker days—as puppets. We might silently wonder what in our daily lives really matters. What genuinely inspires us? Is this all there is?

Does this resonate with you?

Don't beat yourself up if you are an adult who has checked off all the boxes for what it means to be a responsible, successful man, yet you're still dissatisfied.

But until you begin to look at your life differently, ask deeper questions, and take some essential steps, that emptiness will persist and inevitably try to guide you to dark places. It can lead to frustration, anger, resentment, self-pity, and all sorts of destructive choices. You are stuck in a paradox right now: You have a life that you have worked hard to create, but you feel trapped within it and perhaps painfully detached from it. But no matter where you are, there's time to set yourself free, and I suspect now is finally the right time for you.

> **No matter where you are, there's time to set yourself free.**

There are many reasons you might feel like a spectator in your own life, lacking the inner spark that lets you see when all your hard work is meaningful. Sometimes it takes all your effort just to meet your basic needs. Other times, your day is so busy between work and family that there is no room for anything else. Perhaps the most significant factor, however, is the momentum that has built up over the years, as countless small decisions have taken your needs out of the equation in favor of *doing* for everyone else.

The Cost of Success

Success seems predefined in our modern American culture. It guides us toward a one-size-fits-all reward system and nearly always involves the full-time pursuit of money. We participate in this system of success because we want these resources—not only to take care of our families but also to have a status that allows us to move through the world confidently.

However, the act of giving your time in exchange for financial gain is risky—it can easily steal time away from other things in life that are important. I have known plenty of guys who have achieved this coveted financial success many times over. Yet, instead of being excited and present in their lives, they are so focused on making more money they don't seem happy or to be taking advantage of their financial abundance. Even though they have more than enough money to do whatever they want, they seem to hold on tighter than ever, as if the risk of everything falling apart is greater than ever.

Perhaps you wear a mask of cheerfulness in front of your coworkers and family, while inside, you desperately want more. You may even harbor so much resentment that you want to punch a hole in the bedroom wall at night because you've spent your entire day putting out fires for everyone else, and there's no time left for you. Your goal at the end of the day may not be to unwind and relax—maybe you need to escape.

Perhaps you know the frustration that arises when you don't know how to answer the simple question, "How are you doing?" You'd like to say, "How would I know?" because the question feels pointless. "Fine" turns into your go-to response—one that is becoming less and less successful at hiding your building resentment.

Low Expectations

Sadly, many of us operate from a place that's referred to as the *cycle of the middle*. This is defined by coasting in the safe zone, dissatisfied yet not wholly miserable, and successful but not arriving at any destination. You have so much on your plate that keeps you from stepping out and taking risks. You are working so hard to maintain what you have that the idea of change feels overwhelming. You are weighed down by the knowledge that your achievements might only be temporary pleasures, and the prospect of failure scares you to your core. Everything is ready to soak up your energy, time, and money. So, you are just being pulled along by life's currents, letting outside forces make your decisions.

With all that rests on your shoulders, how is there space to discover what you want and need? You're afraid that even asking these questions will make the world you've constructed fall apart. You're worried you will let other people down by prioritizing yourself.

Most of us make decisions based on deeply held beliefs that have been with us for a long time. The world conspires to keep it this way: our conditioning keeps us in our roles and on the most acceptable paths. And many of us find ways to tolerate our suffering. It is not so bad, we tell ourselves. It is our due. We choose to sit in the back seat and let others take risks—and thus reap the rewards. We are somehow okay with all of this. We've found ways to silence ourselves, diminish our potential, uplift those around us, and abandon our well-being.

This burden of low-to-medium expectations that we carry is a form of passivity. It is hard to imagine making different choices because what we do can be so important to those around us. So, we resign ourselves to ignoring our needs. Logic also tells us not to rock the boat since we are checking off many boxes that earn us societal approval. Our willingness to obey can naturally lead us to blame the world for feeling trapped.

We were taught to be team players and play by the rules, and since we tend to do what we are told, we make sure that we are good at it. And because we play the game so well, we believe we should be rewarded with happiness, success, and prosperity. In reality, though, nothing is promised to any of us, and we do ourselves a disservice by defining success in material terms. This dynamic will continue indefinitely until we take responsibility for defining our own needs and desires in this world.

Growing Up

The deep roots of this dilemma can be traced back to childhood. We all have our challenges when we are young. Adults may have the skills and perspective to navigate the struggles that come our way, but children may experience these same difficulties as overwhelming. As kids, we create subconscious strategies to overcome fear, feel safe, and get our needs met. These tactics are inherently neither good nor bad. Their goal is simply to protect us. The issue is the powerful, unseen control they have over us as time goes on. Though we may be in our thirties, forties, fifties, or beyond, these childhood patterns may still be in the driver's seat.

We all have this in common until we finally grow up. And being "a grown-up" has nothing to do with age or how much responsibility you have. A real adult should be defined by their emotional maturity. Becoming emotionally mature means becoming aware of our emotions and letting go of our compulsions to control other people. We come to understand our needs and have the words to express them. We relax into the moment instead of running from crisis to crisis. Having a mature emotional core gives us personal power and guides us to spend our days pursuing more than just what others seek from us. It enables us to explore a more meaningful existence and discover our higher purpose. And though we might believe focusing on our emotional well-being is somehow self-indulgent, in reality, doing so will allow us to create a reality that truly works for us and everyone else in our lives.

Though making fundamental changes might seem like an option you don't have time for, I invite you to let go of that idea. You can discover your wants and desires in simple, straightforward ways so that you see positive results in your daily life. The central aim of this book is to insert new perspectives into your life. We will plant a variety of seeds and watch them grow. The path to personal freedom does not require carving out more time in your day to start a new habit. It does not require that you learn a whole school of thought. At this moment, all that is needed is a willingness to be easier on yourself and give some of your current patterns a rest.

Ultimately, we all want to enjoy our lives and be seen for who we are—not just what we do. That sounds reasonable, yes?

A New View of Success

To be in your power means to be connected to yourself and responsible for your feelings and actions. And it requires acknowledging what might be happening within you. You need to know yourself, what makes you tick, what scares you, and be okay with the good and the bad, the wins and the losses. Be brave enough to look in the mirror. You will discover that the person there is stronger than you realize, a man capable of accomplishing much more than you have imagined.

The good news is that there's a way of being that is much easier and happier than how you may be living now. You can discover many different ways to grow, and they do not require you to reject your current life or give up what you have earned through all your hard work. It is possible to transform your relationship with your life and still hold on to what is essential. You can liberate yourself while still providing for your family or upholding any of the myriad other commitments you want to maintain. It's time to place yourself and your needs squarely at the center of your life and bring out more of the happiness you deserve. It's absolutely within your capabilities to make being your authentic self your default state.

You and I have been doing our best to operate within the societal roles and rules we've assumed as responsible men. The three sections of this book are organized to reflect universal themes of my own experience, foundational for anyone wanting to create change in their life: Awareness, Accountability, and Action. I know personally, viscerally, that trying to navigate life by putting everyone else's needs first leads to pain and a lack of fulfillment. In the hope that my transparency is helpful, I will do my best to own the part I have played in feeling trapped—and in finally finding my way out.

Life is full of responsibilities, and it is entirely possible to have fun carrying them out. It's *how* we show up to our responsibilities that makes the difference. If we are successful financially but burned out from the effort, there may be no satisfaction in having all that cash. It's no wonder we feel empty if we are endlessly busy but have no personal investment in our work.

The pivot from frustration to openness is both simple and subtle. If we are connected to ourselves in the moment so that curiosity about what we're experiencing is front and center, we will be more patient, relaxed, and happy. This new way of being requires that you show up for yourself, first and foremost. By expanding into the uniqueness of who you are, you will begin to live into your new definition of success.

Fellow recovering people pleasers, this book is intended to bring out more of the happiness and freedom that is available to you when you move through your days with a deeper understanding of who you are, what you want, and how to navigate life while expressing your needs with humility and vulnerability. It took me a long time to realize my coping strategies weren't fulfilling or sustainable, but once I decided to illuminate my own needs and desires and better understand how to express them, everything changed for the better. If you, too, are tired of feeling trapped and longing for more meaning in your life, let's begin this journey!

CHAPTER 2

Digging Up the Roots of Dysfunction

A while ago, I found myself in a place where I was making good money, my kids were off at college, and I had survived a divorce. I was suddenly responsible for only myself on a day-to-day level, and my logic told me that this was now "me" time and that everything I had wanted during my years of being responsible for my family was finally going to come my way.

But that didn't happen. I was just as disconnected from myself and unfulfilled as I'd been before. New strains of bitterness and resentment began to show up. All the effort I'd exerted over the years, coupled with societal messages about my privilege and entitlement as a middle-class white man, convinced me that I should be blessed at any moment with that satisfying life I'd been dreaming of.

Since childhood, I have been an introvert, staying in the background of both situations and organizations. Think of me as the quietly competent type. I certainly did not possess the ambition and determination it would take to sell myself or a product when I entered the working world. So my natural way of making a living turned out to be middle management. From there, I could take care of my family's daily needs but not really step up in a way that would help me get ahead. This reality that I chose hid a deep sadness, and my inability to navigate the process of finding more meaningful and sustainable work led me to increasingly numb myself.

Alcohol and porn were overly accessible, naturally self-isolating methods of escape. Because they are so prevalent in our society, it was easy for me to discount these choices as normal dude behavior. But before long, I was feeling emotionally absent across the board. Neither my work nor my personal life gave me a spark. There are cases of depression in my family, and I feared that if I stopped drinking my daily beers, I might slip into that state and feel worse than I already did. At the time, it felt like I might as well just accept that existence generally equated to unhappiness regardless of the specifics. This thinking locked in my malaise. I was afraid of what might happen if I gave up my self-medication more than I hated the suffering it was causing in the present.

Where Unhealthy Strategies Are Born

Floating outside ourselves while we engage in duty after duty, numbing ourselves to suppress the feelings that demand our attention, rationalizing our unhappiness and sense of disconnection: these ways of spending our days don't appear out of nowhere. We all have complicated stories in life, some a mixture of joy and difficulty, others outright damaging.

As men, we are expected to be in command of our emotions and experiences. To keep it all tamped down. There is a fear that it will be too much if we look into the dark corners, and everything will fall apart. But if we are to care for ourselves, we need to address our circumstances and take away the power that buried feelings have over us. Denying our pain leads to layer upon layer of dissociation from ourselves.

When I was in first grade, my teacher asked me to do a writing exercise, and in response, I stabbed the palm of my writing hand with a pencil. Not the outcome she expected, I'm sure, and I didn't seem to have any sort of explanation for this impulse. I also began having migraines and suffered some learning challenges. My parents were doing what they could to support me. I remember counseling and special classes, but there was never any breakthrough or resolution.

At that early age, I was also the smallest kid in class, and I did not start to catch up developmentally until the end of high school. My size, combined with my emotional turmoil, contributed to my becoming very quiet. I blended into the background. In seventh grade, we had to present a book report to the class, and when it was my turn, I froze at the podium and could not speak. My lack of communication was so ever-present that perhaps my defining characteristic was my silence. I even received a special "quiet student" award in class several times during middle school. This encouragement reinforced that living in retreat was the way for me.

In elementary school, my home life also changed. My older brother moved to another state to live with his birth father, and my parents separated a few years later. My mother was busy running her own business, and my father worked primarily out of state for a long time. It felt like everyone went their own way. Our family unit slowly ceased to exist.

> **The emotions we experience as kids can slip into the subconscious.**

Most of us have complex childhoods, and our younger selves can't help but be negatively impacted. The emotions we experience as kids can slip into the subconscious and become part of us, shaping and building our long-term coping strategies. I developed a lifelong tactic of people pleasing. I was a good, quiet boy who did his homework, and that strategy continued into adulthood as I assumed the role of the solid, quiet man who did his job. Little did I know there was a profound, subconscious reason I was conducting my life this way.

When the Unexpected Is Revealed

When I graduated college at age twenty-two, I went back home for the holidays. On New Year's Eve, I answered the phone, and on the other end was someone close to the family calling to wish my mom a happy new year. He was drunk and not expecting to talk to me, so perhaps he was thrown off. Then something happened that I could never have anticipated: after a brief, fumbling conversation, he abruptly confessed that he had sexually molested me when I was five.

When the call ended, I just went about my business numbly. I had repressed the memories so fully that I did not associate what I had just learned with my actual life. But in the days that followed, flashes came back to me, along with disorienting pain and fear. When it happened to me as a child, he told me not to tell anyone. Because he was an authority figure close to my parents, I stayed quiet. I also did not tell anyone because, even though I knew I hadn't done anything wrong, I was riddled with shame.

As I tried to go about navigating my life as a young adult, I began to see how the abuse had impacted me. The source of my "withdrawn nature" was no longer a mystery. I gained more understanding of why I struggled to have lasting relationships with women. I had built walls that would not allow anyone to get close to me.

I mistakenly thought I could move on because I finally knew what had happened to me. Possessing no skills to deal with my pain, I tried to power through. That had seemed to work okay in my life up until that point, and I did not have the awareness to seek any outside help for my new recognition of the abuse. I had a grasp of the facts of my life, but I was still operating from a position of woundedness, so my tendency to retreat remained. I did not understand that knowing about early childhood trauma and its resulting emotional pain is not the same as healing from it.

Living a Double Life

My people-pleasing instincts remained the defining characteristics of my presence in the world. As I had throughout my life, I stayed out of the spotlight and did what was expected of me. Eventually, I opened up to a woman and was able to engage in a longer relationship than anything that had come before. After a couple of years together and the happy surprise of pregnancy, we got married. And once I became a father, I naturally embraced being the provider for my family. I could tie my identity to being that dependable, "do it all" man that society told me I should want to be.

The slowly growing obstacle I faced, one entirely invisible to me, was that I was living a double life. On the inside, I was still a scared, wounded child who wanted nothing more than to be left alone, while on the outside, I was a husband, father, and working adult racing through his days to fulfill requirements. Each of these aspects was significant enough on its own to dominate my experience. Unfortunately, they were also wholly incompatible.

I felt overwhelmed all the time. Without having learned healthy ways to manage my feelings or express my needs, I was working desperately to maintain a life that was wearing me out. While I wasn't aware of this deeper pain overshadowing me, I knew I was beginning to feel imprisoned.

The Only Way Out Is Through

My life revolved around a long list of priorities, and I was nowhere on that list. My strategies for managing pain and frustration had not changed much since I was in college. The man was older, but the boy was still in charge.

I saw my growing habit of drinking beer as "me" time (like many of you, I know how easily coping mechanisms intertwine with destructive behavior). I would stop and buy beer on the way home from work and drink it while cooking or helping with kids' homework. I so undervalued myself that I thought this was the best version of "me" time I deserved. After all, I told myself, there was no time for me because of all my responsibility, so I had better take advantage of the cold beer in my hand to enjoy myself.

There were periods when I maintained some balance, but those were overshadowed by the many other times I drank to excess.

The compulsion always came back to the need to numb all the thoughts and feelings in my head and—at least for a moment—escape my life. This pattern continued for years. I knew that my drinking and growing resentment and disconnection harmed myself and those around me, but I could not find a way to feel happy without it. My connection with my wife suffered, and so did my relationship with my children. When I ultimately decided to leave the marriage, I worried about the impact on my kids. Parenting felt like a minefield of ways I might already be harming my kids, and I didn't want to drop the trauma of divorce on them. But my sense of being trapped was becoming unbearable, and I thought that changing my circumstances would give me the freedom and happiness I craved.

From my current perspective, I see I was running away from a situation more than running toward myself. Decades after childhood, I was still watching my life unfold passively without being directly engaged.

After divorce, my increasing sorrow led me into depression and to reach for ways to suppress it, which looped back to sadness and self-pity so that my emotions fed on themselves like the snake eating its tail.

I saw myself as a "doer." I was a paycheck, an employee, a consumer, and another person just passing through the days. And when my friends or my own thoughts encouraged me to address my problems, I inevitably failed. It took me more years than I wish it had to realize that changes weren't happening because I was only trying to please the people who had asked for them.

During one wasted morning spent hung over, the sourness of my self-loathing behavior crystallized into the understanding that I was making decisions as if I wasn't even worth my own time. Like I didn't deserve my effort. The clarity of this felt like a fist to the face. I had arrived at a place where I could no longer accept my excuses.

Reclamation

I had to make a change. I imagined my life continuing the way it was, and all I could see was a flat, featureless landscape. My core experiences seemed to revolve around sitting at a desk and then trying to drink the boredom away at night. Wash, rinse, repeat. A sense that life is pointless had been gaining too much traction in my mind, and that scared me deeply.

Many of my middle-aged male peers were hitting this wall as well. Around this time, three men I knew took their lives. Perhaps it was the loss of friends that knocked some sense into me. I was not happy or thriving; I did not have a purpose that felt deeply powerful and true. I needed meaning.

Action was required. I chose the most obvious example of how I had been banging my head on the wall for so long. I stopped drinking. It had already gone too far, and I did not want to discover what would happen should it worsen. This was a huge first step in prioritizing myself. And when I removed the substance I'd been using to numb myself, I finally had the clarity of mind and courage to work on my issues.

Sobriety would come to open many doors both directly and indirectly: I found love, connected more intimately with my kids, and was brave enough to start a company as I learned to identify and chase my dreams.

Looking deeper, though, this practical decision to stop drinking was the outcome of a bold yet quietly whispered decision: to put myself first without exception. To love myself and learn to know that I am worthy of this love. Quitting drinking did not solve all my problems, but it set the stage to create lasting, positive change in my life.

And so, I embraced the fact that if I wanted to be happy, I had to be my own most important priority. I needed to question my assumptions about how I lived. I needed to stop being passive. I chose to be brave enough to let go of a self that was forged from the collection of roles I had assumed. Instead, I resolved to see myself thoroughly, with curiosity and fresh eyes.

The Path Forward

I found a skilled therapist who helped me address my wounding, and I learned that the challenges I faced in my adult life were not random things that happened to me, nor were they predetermined by the roles I chose. I saw that the strategies I'd used to endure my inner pain had led to my choices and their outcomes. In later chapters, we will dig into how our deepest (and often hidden) emotions are expressed in our decision-making. For now, know that all of us must navigate our inner experience if we desire more freedom and happiness and that, with some intention, this inner reflection can teach us a lot and show us what's really important in life.

> **All of us must navigate our inner experience if we desire more freedom and happiness.**

For me, growth has come mainly from being able to look at my different aspects and neither rejecting nor fearing what I see. My issues are interesting to me now that they no longer have me tied up in knots. As I accepted that there was a *me* inside that deserved to be set free, my confidence began to increase. Absorbing the reality that *I am more than what I do in the world and that I am not a victim of circumstances*, I have come to see that the fears that held so much influence over me and determined most of my choices were just stories I told myself. As I faced and named them, I saw that they only had the power I gave them.

Being passive does not mean that we have no responsibility for what happens. Passivity is a way of managing painful experiences when we don't have other techniques. I had to become proactive and take ownership of everything I manifested, the good and the bad. This simple, earth-shaking shift in attitude would result in a much more exciting and gratifying existence.

> **Passivity is a way of managing painful experiences when we don't have other techniques.**

This can happen for you as well. You can liberate yourself when you take responsibility for your happiness with the same vigor you've brought to so many other roles in your life. Acknowledging that change is up to us may feel overwhelming, but that sensation can be quickly replaced by the relief of knowing how easy actual change can be. That's right, *easy*.

We stay small and stuck when we don't ask questions and when we assume that how things are is how they will always be. I want to shake you, wake you up, and tell you that transformation is possible! You and I have shown how capable we are at managing burdens on behalf of others. Let's take those skills and apply them to our own experiences, our own intelligence, and our own strengths. Let's use what we've devoted to the outside world to bring lasting meaning to our own lives.

Onward and Upward

Loving yourself enough to put your happiness at the top of your list of responsibilities is not an intellectual exercise. There is no rationalizing or coercing or justifying. When we say the words "I love myself," we must back them up with actions to prove that it is true. We may find it easy to say that we love our family and friends, but we men find it much more challenging to direct love toward ourselves. There is also no shame in it. But when we are disconnected from ourselves, expressing that emotion can feel stupid or forced. Does it feel natural to say "I love you" to yourself right now? Do you believe it when you say it?

Loving ourselves is not something another person can gift us. No one's approval will kindle the flame. We have no option but to create that change for ourselves. As I did it for myself, I began to experience life from a place of deep and strong emotions instead of always trying to be cerebral. Our minds are great tools for strategizing and getting things done, but we must rely on our hearts for newer and more profound understanding, connection, and happiness.

The Time Is Now

It is never too late to change and heal, just like it's never pointless to care. I am in my early fifties and thrilled with where my life has ventured. I do not look back and wish that things had been different. I've found that it's better to put that mental effort into building a life that makes me happy today. This is the big picture: the present moment. Our work together does not call for regret over the past or stress about the future. In the following chapters, from a place of our shared experience, I'll share simple steps to help you break free from the trap you're in and help you actively build the meaningful life you've been searching for.

CHAPTER 3

○○○ — — — ○○○

Healthier, Happier, and More Present

"Personal growth lies within the unknown;
courage permits you to explore this space."

—Unknown

Suffering can range from dramatic to silent, but it is almost always in charge when it is present. I know a practical way through this suffering to a more fulfilling relationship with yourself and more contentment and ease as you navigate your life, which I'll share in the following chapters of this book. It took me a long time to understand that we aren't alone in our struggles and that many others can understand and relate to us when we are brave enough to share what we are going through. Though our stories differ, by sharing mine, I hope you can see that you are not alone in your desire for personal freedom.

> **We aren't alone in our struggles.**

Easeful Exploration

While the broader purpose of this book is to share practices that have helped me arrive at a healthier, happier, and more present place, my real aim is to give you simple, straightforward suggestions for connecting with yourself and improving your life. It's remarkable how seeing yourself in new ways can naturally build on itself and become habituated.

We men who identify mainly as providers and doers find ourselves deeply entrenched in predictable roles. Many of the tasks we perform are essential in handling the practical aspects of life. Others have to do with relationships and behavioral patterns. The prompts outlined in this book will allow you to make significant changes without having to upend your entire life.

To maintain what's good and working in our lives while we engage in transformation, we must embody the knowledge that the most important relationship to change is our relationship with ourselves. Our relationships with others and with our daily experiences will naturally shift once we build this foundational connection to ourselves. When we prioritize our connection to ourselves, change becomes easier because we know where to put our energy.

> **The most important relationship to change is our relationship with ourselves.**

Importantly, I want to define what I mean when I say *connection* because you will see this word a lot. For the purpose of this book, connection with yourself means:

- Being curious about what makes you tick
- Knowing what you need to take care of yourself and doing it
- Not backing away from personal challenges
- Being open and excited about what is to come

I encourage you to add whatever other statements you find reflect directly on what it means to feel connected to yourself. How you learn is individual to you, and after reading this book, you should be able to adapt (and add to) these simple tools so that your sense of connection to yourself is tailored to who you are and what you want out of your life.

And on that note, let's talk about the words we choose to use when engaging with ourselves. Let's be positive, encouraging, *and* pragmatic. Train yourself out of seeing your glass as half empty. The heaviness we feel when negative words circulate in our minds weighs us down, reduces creativity, and makes it much harder to improve our lives.

For example, though it's used commonly, I do not resonate with referring to personal growth or healing as "work" or even "the good work." In my experience, work is the place where we perform tasks and receive compensation. When I hear people talk about this inner journey as some sort of "personal work," it drains my desire to go there. I don't want more work! I do not want to feel that I must make more time in my schedule to engage in some new obligation. You may have a different relationship with this term, of course. The important thing is that you pay attention to the emotional resonance of the language you use.

Are there any terms that make you cringe or shut you down? There are others that do that for me, but I don't want to color your experience with my hang-ups! Let's agree to choose our words wisely. Use language that encourages and inspires you to move from Point A to Point B and then steadily onward.

How This Book Is Organized

During my most challenging times, I wondered what it would be like to have faith, to have the conviction that whatever was happening was ultimately good and that something out there had my back. Spiritually speaking, I am attracted to certain aspects of different religions and philosophies. Holding this perspective allows me to wander where my interests take me, which is a great thing. The difficulty is that lacking a foundational belief system has made me feel like I was missing something important.

I realized that if there were to be a core framework to my beliefs, I would need to create my own path to understand myself, heal my wounds, and elevate my daily experience. And because I like to think through and straightforwardly organize things, I hope my process and how I've organized this book will resonate with you.

The book is organized into three distinct sections and further divided by specific themes, which you'll learn about next. The book's first two sections focus on our minds and emotions and how our inner experiences inform our outer lives. The third section is about nurturing our drive to create a life that reflects our uniqueness and potential. Each section offers practical observations, insights, and suggestions.

In each section, you will find simple contemplations and exercises to do and reflect upon. The practices in this book are designed to invoke curiosity and fun so that all your daily experiences are richer. Consider keeping a notebook and pen on hand and making time to engage with these prompts. Writing down ideas and feelings allows us to try them out in a more profound way than by simply thinking about them. Think of writing down a thought as committing to it just a little. You will quickly see what feels true and what doesn't.

Section I: Awareness

Awareness comes first because it's the foundation upon which everything else is built. This is the section that I equate most with our thinking minds. We need to trust ourselves and our decision-making—and cultivate awareness about why we behave the way we do—to have a healthy operating system.

Three Steps to Awareness:

- Chapter 4: Respect the Life that You Have Built – Though you are embarking on a transformation of sorts, it's important that you recognize the gifts and strengths you already possess. In this chapter, you are guided through exercises to help you own the successes you've already achieved.
- Chapter 5: Question Your Assumptions – Your ways of seeing your life and the methods you use to navigate it started out as ways to help you stay safe. But now they may be causing you to stay stuck. This chapter digs into our self-limiting views and how to remove our blinders.
- Chapter 6: Observe What's Present – Meaningful change cannot happen unless it is rooted in personal truth. This chapter challenges you to look in the mirror and be honest with yourself about how you currently navigate the world.

Section II: Accountability

The title of this section may trigger a little bit of stress in you. Accountability, after all, is one of the aspects of our lives that has put us in this position of overload. Yet, while it is important to be accountable to those we love, we also have a duty to be authentic and accountable to ourselves—expressing our deepest desires, talents, and a sense of purpose. As we foster more happiness and satisfaction within, we'll have more inner peace, which will go on to impact others positively.

Accountability is also a helpful tool when taking on a new goal. Let's step out of our usual perspective and shift our attention to what is inside us as we explore the direct power of *personal accountability*.

Three Steps to Accountability:

- Chapter 7: Own Your Power – Many of us imagine we are the victims of cruel, external forces. This belief, while possibly self-supportive, can also be immobilizing. In this chapter, you will have the opportunity to change your view of yourself from a person who is passive to one who is engaged.
- Chapter 8: Face Your Fears – This chapter invites you to do what every one of us dreads: face what frightens you. With exercises and a slice of my recent history, I will accompany you through this process. It's very liberating to discover that it is in facing what scares us that we can most easily be released from its power.
- Chapter 9: Open Up to Connection – Many of us have spent years, even decades, disconnected from our true feelings, wishes, and needs. This chapter makes the case that to be intimate with other people and the world around us, we must first forge a connection to ourselves. Questions and exercises offer a pathway to begin that process.

Section III: Action

This book's final section takes us deeper into the changes we seek. It requires that you know that you are worth this effort. Then, it's a matter of stepping up and claiming your worth to get where you want to go.

Action is about taking tangible, achievable steps. And it's 100 percent your responsibility. Though that might seem like daunting news to you, you will get to a place where this fact is empowering. You are fully capable of making changes, and the more you take charge of your happiness instead of outsourcing it to other people, the more likely it is that you will reach your state of bliss.

Three Steps to Action:

- Chapter 10: Create Momentum – The steps that we take to improve our lives do not happen in a vacuum. Though we may feel that events unfold randomly, we can shift our perspective to create coherence and build confidence.
- Chapter 11: Explore Your Purpose – Unleashing your true self alters how you approach your daily life. It provides much-deserved contentment and a newfound sense of agency. Before long, you may find yourself seeking something bigger, a guiding light, an organizing principle. In this chapter, we will discuss your higher aims, and you'll identify what you value most and explore the creation of a personal mission statement.
- Chapter 12: Ever-Expanding You – The book concludes with this chapter that reminds you of the

> power of your struggle for liberation and the magic of its rewards. You have navigated some challenging inner exploration. Of course, the journey continues. But you are engaged in the process of setting yourself free, and that is cause for celebration.

Honest Truth

As you move through the coming pages, be open to shifting your definition of strength. When you face hard truths within you, honor yourself for your openness to taking a leap into new perspectives.

> **Be open to shifting your definition of strength.**

Creating lasting change is not always easy. It requires that we address our deeply held strategies and perspectives. Get ready to be honest with yourself. The process asks us to gather our lives in our hands and take responsibility for how we experience it. What you want cannot occur without trading some comfort for risk and the trance of passivity for action. Each action you take will beget another and another, and you may find that focusing on transformation becomes a pleasure.

SECTION 1

AWARENESS

CHAPTER 4

ooo— — —ooo

Respect the Life That You Have Built

As we embark on this journey together, I want to invite you to take a step back from your productivity and responsibilities for a moment and take a broader view of your life. Can you see how much you have accomplished and how powerful you already are? Knowing you have the capability and strength to make positive changes in your life is essential. And that change does not require capsizing everything or starting over from scratch. Transformation begins when you better understand your choices and the patterns that guide them.

Ultimately, we want to see what is going on for us at any given moment so we can be present and not react automatically. To move toward that goal, we must recognize and affirm the excellent foundation that is already in place. This will help us develop a healthy and well-earned baseline of respect for ourselves.

> It's crucial to find the value in what you do.

It's crucial to find the value in what you do. More than likely, you are actively engaged in the world, even if you want to run from it in difficult circumstances. You are a survivor who gets things done. It's important to see it all because the full picture—including every beautiful event, large and small—is made up of the moments of your life. And your participation in your own life is worth your appreciative attention. We all have deep reserves to help handle whatever comes our way, and this inner strength can help us ignite the power to create the changes we most want to see.

You in the World

Because you have been able to achieve a great deal, there is no doubt that you can do more to raise the upper limit on your expectations—and do so with intentionality and precision. Accessing this expanded ability is a multistep process that will benefit from some exploration. Let's start by focusing on some of your big accomplishments in order to recognize your efforts as the victories they are.

Self-Reflection

First, identify and write down a list of ten accomplishments that you have achieved, things that would qualify as "foundational." These are the big ones like graduating college, getting an important job or degree, getting married, starting a family, buying a house, excelling at a sport or activity, getting a raise or promotion, learning how to play an instrument, moving cross-country, etc. In other words, this list is about the mountains you have climbed. Spend no more than ten minutes on the list, and if you run out of steam before then, don't worry about it. Keep the list handy over the next week so you can build it out as more accomplishments come to mind.

How did writing this list land for you? Was it a smooth experience, or did you start to trail off around number five, like I did when

I first tried this exercise? If so, that's just fine. When I make a list of any sort, I tend to rattle off a few obvious things and then go blank. Try slowing down or even stepping away. Go about your day with this prompt in the back of your mind. More accomplishments will come to you. Make sure to add them in writing.

There are two reasons for doing this inventory in a way that can gradually build upon itself. The first is that we want to be kind to ourselves and not feel discouraged if, at this time, we cannot fill out a complete roster of our accomplishments. The other reason is that, by sitting with the list and letting it fill out over time, we are creating new thought patterns around the positive aspects of our experience. It's about making space to see ourselves in more profound and different ways and then making it a habit. This deeper perspective will feel good, and we may quickly find that this encouraging view of our life becomes more regular in our daily experiences.

Let's now get a little more granular. Every day is filled with wins, whether you can see them or not, and it's crucial to consider these details as you come to appreciate the enormity of all you get done. Here are some ideas to get the process flowing. This exercise, even more than the previous one, will likely gather momentum once you get into the flow. Remember, your actions have value, including the ones you might dismiss as minor or routine.

Self-Reflection

List ten things you did last week that support the structure of your life: maybe cooking for family, socializing with friends, resolving a disagreement with your partner, fixing a broken cabinet door that had been bugging you for months, or walking the dog every morning. What's happening in your days? The point is to understand that these actions are worthy of your attention. Let's get to a place where we can respect even the chores because *we took the time to do them.* They reflect how you are already connected to and in charge of your life.

After you get through ten items, or however many feel right, I encourage you to expand the timeframe to a month and then come up with another batch of good stuff you've done.

The Horizon Expands

One reason to look at these lists is that we need to incorporate longer timelines into our perspective. If we get caught up in the issues of the moment, we feel stuck in the thorny weeds. We feel immersed in the smaller, immediate tasks (a.k.a. chores) and lack a healthy perspective on the overall picture. In that place, all problems tend to feel intractable, and all requirements on our time overwhelming. But in taking note of our big breakthroughs, as well as those seemingly insignificant daily tasks, we can begin to see the big picture: we are strong, we are diligent, and we regularly manifest what we choose to make happen.

There are times when the world requires meaningful action from us and times when it hammers us with constant smaller demands. We can create space for all of life's requests and needs while also being our own rock. Once we begin to rest on this foundation of healthy perspectives and respect for our skills and experience, we can create a centered life where we are our greatest priority while also connecting to and supporting others.

> **We can create space for all of life's requests and needs while also being our own rock.**

This shift in perception will help you accept life as it happens and make the necessary changes to position yourself as the lead character in your new story.

CHAPTER 5

○○○— — —○○○

Question Your Assumptions

We know that we are here to live out our uniqueness and be all we can be, yet there does not seem to be space to dream up a higher vision for ourselves. To determine what more is possible, we must examine our current assumptions and strategies and learn how to catch ourselves when we are ambling through our days on autopilot. In that unconscious mode, we rely on our assumptions about ourselves and others to make decisions that keep us stuck in our ruts. Our perspective shrinks, and we operate in a constant state of fight or flight. Our inner voice can become silenced, replaced with the always audible needs of work and family.

Questioning our assumptions makes sense on the path toward personal change. When we are open to the idea that what we've been doing is not working, unlocking our potential becomes easier. And letting up on our need to be in control allows us to raise our gaze from our tasks and take in what's around us. If we can be both curious and brave in this process, we can make rapid progress in connecting to ourselves in a way that lessens our general sense of frustration and offers a welcome sense of expansion.

Misguided Assumptions

As responsible guys, we often behave as *we think* others want us to, but we are typically not present enough to take the full situation into account. I know I was too busy "helping" to slow down and consider whether my actions were actually useful. That responsibility train sped along so fast that I couldn't get off. That meant I didn't have to think about whether I was even on the right track. That last bit was especially scary because even entertaining the notion that I was on the wrong track risked opening the door to the belief that everything had been a waste of time and effort.

Guided by the assumptions we've been programmed to hold, many of us try to be the man we think everyone expects of us. We pursue and acquire things that might feel good in the moment but only end up cluttering our garage, literally or metaphorically. We act as caretakers for those around us, viewing our efforts as invaluable, even when others are perfectly capable of handling their own affairs. If we are to wrestle ourselves free, we *must* change the assumption that our value is determined by what we do in the world and what we have acquired.

> **We *must* change the assumption that our value is determined by what we do in the world.**

A few guideposts have emerged for me through the process of asking my own questions. I offer them here as encouragement to pay attention to the personal truths that begin to arise for you:

- Our relationships will not change until we change.
- Our potential will not be fulfilled until we see the part we play in our suffering.

- Once we confront our role in the challenges we've experienced, we can identify what things are in our power to change.
- The path forward is much clearer when we are not lost in the stories we tell ourselves about our experiences.

For me, revisiting these statements brings a sense of ease because they remind me of both the power and the responsibility that I bring to a situation. They are also humble reminders that I must care about myself and prioritize my experience so that I will be more likely to engage with the world in a healthy and mature way. They help make it less likely that I will be my own worst enemy.

Safe and Boring

When I was deep in self-pity, holding down my job felt like as much ambition as I could handle. Stray dreams that floated by in my mind were suppressed by the unceasing pressure to show up and work. On a very practical level, I thought I should be satisfied with any decent employment that provided for my family's needs. At least, that is the message I had to hammer home to myself every day, especially on Sundays.

You know how weekends are: the time when we would *like* to downshift into a quieter, slower gear when we *should* get to do things that align more with our desires. For me, Sunday was not that day. Oh, the day was great for about an hour after waking. But after that, the caffeine had settled in, my brain was fully awake, and thoughts of the work week ahead started to intrude. My mood for each Sunday was wrecked by knowing that Monday was to follow.

Early in my adult life, so much of my value and identity was tied up in being a worker, and I thought that anything more profound I might do in the world would have to be tied to my work. Yet, my drive to succeed was mixed with that fear and passivity that kept me in the background. This meant that I was hoping for outside forces to make sure that I was fulfilled.

Though living this way felt miserable, there was an upside. I knew how to make ends meet, and that's a terrific survival skill. Unfortunately, I viewed sheer survival as my baseline standard for success.

By living in the "safe middle," we hope to dodge problems and limit our struggles. But operating in this way also means that we will not get to explore our deep desires for more meaning and purpose in life.

Turning the Corner

Why does this life seem rigged against me? A version of that question has likely crossed your mind at some point. When things seem unfair, our suffering is rooted in the feeling that something is being imposed upon us. No one likes being told what to do, and yet we live in a society where so many things are decided for us before we even realize that choices are available.

It took hitting rock bottom to understand how fundamentally I needed to reshape my thinking around what I experienced as victimhood. And instead of expecting some life-altering epiphany, I gave myself the gift of taking incremental steps. I simply began to ask myself the questions in this book. The more I did so, the more patient I became with myself and the more curious

I got about what might be revealed. Showing basic curiosity about why we do what we do is a radical gesture that pushes back against automatic behavior and passivity. Taking things one step at a time also allowed me to allay my fears that my life would all fall apart if I examined it too closely. One simple action led to another; understanding one perspective shed light on another; each outdated strategy questioned and released made room for something new.

> **Showing basic curiosity about why we do what we do is a radical gesture.**

I needed to assess the path I was on and figure out where I had let others take over and determine my course of action. This examination was not about blaming anyone. There is such a rapid and connected flow to life that if you are not making decisions for yourself, there are always others ready to make them for you. And when you allow others to dictate the terms of your engagement, then the things you take on will probably match neither your abilities nor your potential.

Self-Reflection

As you look more closely at the lack of satisfaction in your life, I invite you to reflect on the following questions about a particular role you are fulfilling. Perhaps start with a role that may feel tedious or tiring but is not the biggest obstacle to your happiness. Like sitting on a committee that doesn't interest you, serving as the family taxi, tracking budgets and paying bills, caretaking pets or elders in the family—you get the idea.

- What is one role you are fulfilling that you feel was assigned to you by someone else?
- What is that role providing you and those in your life?
- What is it costing you in terms of time? How about energy?
- Can you identify the steps that placed you in this situation? What did you do or not do that allowed it to develop?
- How do you feel about performing this role?
- Do your efforts provide a clear benefit?
- Does dissatisfaction or frustration show up in how you communicate with others or fulfill your role?

Asking and answering these questions can help us get to the heart of personal responsibility by seeing how we give ourselves away.

Think about the situation that you identified above. Likely, in that case and others, your decisions (or indecision) led to the tendency to keep your head down without seeing where you are headed. This kind of passivity is fundamental to feeling trapped in our lives.

When we ask why we do what we do, the very act of questioning loosens the grip of our no-longer-constructive strategies. We can begin to believe that there is no one way to do things. We can invite more inquisitiveness and creativity as we assess our lives and imagine what is possible. By examining the roles that we have chosen to play, we can open the door to essential and profound resets.

CHAPTER 6

○○○— — —○○○

Observe What's Present

As my story proves, we can spend decades cycling through the same unhealthy patterns. Details change, but the big picture is likely to be the same. In my own life, the tactics I developed at a young age remained in control well into adulthood without my knowledge of their existence. Performing as a father and provider easily consumed the time and energy I had available. Family and careers can be beautiful, but when we allow them to own our experience, we fall into a rut that locks us out of discovering what lights us up from the inside out.

Over the years, this rut becomes our world. The barriers to escape get higher, and an awareness of other ways of being gets cloudier. When I realized that nothing was coming to my rescue, that I would not be able to cash in just because I played the game, I felt cornered and out of options. I wanted to lash out but couldn't risk blowing up the structure that was providing for my family and me. The only one I could get away with blaming was the person in the mirror, and so, out of resentment for where I found myself, I became my own worst enemy.

Looking in the Mirror

When it came to my perceived powerlessness, I found it easiest to blame others—not just people in my personal life but people all the way up the scale, from employers to the government. Everyone and everything seemed designed to hold me back. This sense of injustice gave me the excuse to wallow in my anger and feed my demons. It also gave me the excuse to shrink back and not do things that might make a difference in my life.

When we are suffering, placing blame on external forces may feel convenient, but it is one of the most disempowering decisions we can make. Happiness and connectedness to our experience will not fully develop if we fixate on outside forces that we perceive to be failing us. Yes, people will disappoint us or cause us problems, just as we are sure to do to others. Humans are imperfect, and society is messy. But when our expectations require "others" to behave in a certain way to make us feel good, we are likely to end up frustrated and unhappy.

I believe we are here for a reason: We each have specific things to learn and purposes to fulfill. Deep down, when we expect to be handed something because we've played by the rules of society, we are ultimately looking for shortcuts and shying away from our potential. Does it serve us in this life to be handed our victories?

My ego had worked so hard and for so long, but I finally reached the point where even I had to call bullshit on myself. I could see that I was in charge of my life in only the most cursory, practical ways. I was worn out, and weeks of rest or a spectacular vacation would not cure me. It took prolonged personal suffering and denial for me to see the snare in which I was caught.

Society had trained me well to believe it was selfish to prioritize my needs over those of others. I was the eternal pleaser, helping until it hurt. But it is not rational to think we can give endlessly without any thought to refilling the tank.

> Putting yourself first is a process.

When I eventually had nothing left to give, I became open to adding myself to my list of priorities and to putting myself right at the top. A responsible guy will often exhaust himself from doing things for others before he can see that something is not right. Putting yourself first is a process, though, especially if you've been slogging through your days devoted to everyone else's needs.

Examining Your Feelings

Taking your first steps to deepen your awareness takes real courage. I mean that. Once you see yourself beyond the mask you wear for the world, you have entered a powerful part of your journey.

And so, let's take another step forward with some mental exercises. The following method of taking personal inventory may feel clunky at first, but don't worry. The process can be revisited and built upon, and new information will always be available to you. As fresh challenges in life arise, you will likely find yourself creating questions that get to the heart of your unique experience. This prompt is designed to open the door to your feelings. Though our difficult emotions may be muted or locked away, we must begin to identify and process them. Writing them down allows us to wrap our heads around them and diffuse their unseen influence—and with the mental space we clear, we can finally perceive the beauty that already exists in front of us. After the exercise, if you want to tear up the paper or delete the file, feel free! It is perfectly fine to leave no evidence of your thoughts as they try to take shape. As we move through this book, I want you to feel safe and confident that no one is looking over your shoulder. This is very important because your connection to yourself will be hindered if you are somehow trying to take someone else's opinion into account.

Self-Reflection

Get some paper and answer the following questions honestly. This exercise is designed to help you get in touch with your challenging emotions:

- What makes you angry? Write about any topics that call to you. You don't have to focus on something you aren't ready to face—but it is crucial that you let yourself feel at least a bit of discomfort. If it is easier, start with an issue at work instead of your personal life.
- Once you have a few items, go to the one that rises most in your thoughts. What are the things about this situation that make you angry? What is it that you want to happen here that isn't happening?
- How might you be contributing to this situation?
- Assume that you can't change the behavior of others. By focusing on your own decisions, what actions might you take so that you experience less suffering in this situation?

Exploring your emotions on the page can help you consider the feeling from different angles. Sit with the feeling and see how it fits into your broader experience. Is this feeling something that is stirred up in many circumstances? Do you sense any other emotions that come with it? Have you felt disrespected or used? What happened? Remember, right now, we are not trying to solve a problem. We are simply practicing sitting with an emotion so that we can name it and understand how it's wrapped into our daily lives.

Playing the Part

Regarding the experience of the challenging emotion, you may feel that it takes your senses over completely and causes stress from head to toe. Per the example above, you may not know where the anger begins and where it ends, which is normal. So, in the moment, this emotion defines your experience. To better navigate powerful, difficult emotions, we need to organize our thoughts in a way that holds emotions, so they can be examined and addressed without taking us over. In my case, I underwent a process called parts work with my psychotherapist (see Additional Resources at the back of the book for more information).

Briefly, parts work asks us to go back to the first time we remember an emotion being present in our lives. We do not have to relive a bad experience; we just want to understand the context in which the feeling arose. At that point, we can engage with the part of ourselves at the age we were when the event occurred. That part of us is holding on to the memory and emotion, and by imagining we are meeting it as an adult, we see what we can do to move the feeling through and toward release. That way, this old emotion is no longer where our brains go when a similar stressful situation arises.

This has been effective for me because, instead of just dealing with the present-day thing that triggered my anger or other emotions, the parts work helped me identify the root cause of the feeling. With parts work, we can remain present in the moment at hand instead of retreating into old patterns of emotional pain.

> **With parts works, we can remain present in the moment at hand instead of retreating into old patterns.**

In chapter 2, I recounted how I stabbed my hand in the first grade when my teacher asked me to do something. It was an impulsive act that involved no planning or forethought. What was that anger communicating? Ultimately, I learned that it had its roots in abuse, but that level of understanding is not required to engage with the feelings that were present. As an adult in this new context of parts work, my goal was to pause, observe, and engage with that younger part of myself—not to relive the anger but also not to shy away from the fact that it was there.

When I slowed down and sat with this memory, I saw that the younger part of me had the desire to reject the world of adults. Honestly, it's a feeling that makes a lot of sense coming from a child, considering how much chaos we adults tend to create. By seeing that stabbing my hand was this younger self's way of saying he was angry, I validated his experience and felt more connected to this time in my life. I could feel a loosening inside myself as the memory changed from this random, wild lashing out to a more understandable expression of fear—perhaps the only type of expression a confused child could manage. This personal understanding was soothing. My connection to my experience deepened. I felt more at peace thanks to helping that younger part of me feel seen and understood.

Self-Reflection

And so, when you feel ready—now, tomorrow, or next week—take time to answer the following questions. This internal dialogue I'm asking you to engage in may feel funny, but please stick with it!

- Can you recall a time in your childhood when you first experienced anger?
- Can you feel a connection to this younger part of yourself?
- What would this younger version of yourself like to tell you about why he feels angry?
- Can you understand where he's coming from?
- Can you let him know your adult self is here with him now and tell him it's safe for him to let you know he's mad and that you're in this together?
- Can you, as the adult, tell him you've got his back? Because if you can, you should.

Balancing Our Perspectives

As you learn to examine some of your deeper emotions, let's balance things out a little by taking in the view of where you are right now. What are some hard-earned perspectives that you can access to navigate your life? Personal wisdom is coursing through you right now, and it's available when we can slow down and name it. Trust me when I tell you that amazing things can happen for you at this stage, even before you can see the larger road map ahead.

> **We do not have to transform everything at once to feel better about our lives.**

As examples, here are a few helpful truisms that presented themselves to me on my path of self-care. Even though everything in this list exists elsewhere in some other form, when I began to mull these concepts over after committing to caring about myself, they all felt like new territory to explore. And because they are worded in my own style, they have greater sticking power for when I need a higher, more balanced perspective on my life.

- If something in our lives needs to change, it is up to us to make it happen.
- When we are resentful, angry, defensive, numb, or generally in escape mode, our awareness of what might be happening in a situation is limited, and our ability to get through it productively is almost nil.
- When we are stuck in an unhealthy pattern of behavior, change can feel impossible.
- When we question our assumptions about our role in things, we are automatically less passive and more likely to get away from a sense of victimhood.
- We can be okay with the fact that we cannot do it all. In fact, we can be overjoyed to know that we should not even try!

- When our connection to ourselves is solid, we can make decisions that are in our best interest and do not come at the expense of others.
- By reflecting on our experiences, we are strengthening one of our most essential resources for change: our hard-earned perspective.
- We do not have to transform everything at once to feel better about our lives.

Connecting to these few broad, personal truths expanded the cracks in my armor so a little more light could shine in. A logic, a basicness, to these ideas calmed me. The statements stood on their own, did not rely on anyone else for success, and didn't attach themselves to some desired future. It would be premature to say that I had already achieved a genuine connection to myself, but at least I was learning to challenge my assumptions about how unfair life was. I was also feeling a little more space inside of me. Less tension and constriction. More room for my voice.

It may seem counterintuitive to find comfort in questioning our perspectives and decisions, but that is the door we must pass to leave behind our self-destructive ways. It is also the point at which we begin to understand how complex and powerful we really are. And feeling our worth is at the heart of feeling safe and at ease. It offers us the deepest kind of comfort.

What Do You Deserve?

Next, let's touch on passivity and entitlement. When we think we deserve something just because we've played by the rules, we are lighting a long fuse of resentment. We are not guaranteed anything in this life, and it will not be pretty when the fuse burns all the way down, and our emotions finally ignite.

That being said, society dangles countless dreams and versions of success in front of us, and our egos hungrily latch onto those that best fit our vision for ourselves. It's hard not to want what others have achieved, and if it happened for these other people, then it's past time for us to get ours! Let's examine how we latch onto expectations for success and happiness. If we assume that these great things will appear in our lives, but we are not actively planning or working on making them happen, this may be a sign that we are operating from a sense of entitlement.

Self-Reflection

When we set goals or establish dreams, we want to attach them to existing or attainable skills and achievable effort. When we think that something will happen for us simply because of who we are, we sell ourselves short and limit the depth of experience we could have by pursuing these goals through our own effort and inspiration.

- Be honest about what you have felt you deserve over time. What successes have you expected to be handed that weren't?
- Why did that goal seem accessible to you even though it may have been outside your daily experience or long-term planning? Were you counting on family support to get you there? Was it something promised via higher education? Was it a goal you started but did not take the time to see to the end? In other words, who was going to rescue you by making your dream a reality?

- How do you respond when these dreams and goals don't manifest for you? Do you reflect on what you could do better, or do you tend to assign blame to the situation and other people?
- What happens if you focus on reasons for your disappointments that have to do with your own actions or inaction? Make space to see how your choices have helped shape your outcomes.
- Do you find yourself experiencing resistance to seeing your actions through this lens of personal responsibility? Sit with the sensation. Write down what's on your mind to encourage more thoughts and awareness. Note what feels true versus what might be excuses you've been making for yourself.

Tell the truth. Listen for it and hear it when it rises inside you. Be brave and uncompromising. There is no need to get the words all just right. You do not need to be careful to frame things to be fair or protective. This exercise is meant to prime you to connect with who you are and what you want. When that happens, many of your worries about fairness will fall away because you will be operating from a place that supports you and those around you.

There will likely come a time when you will benefit from outside, professional support. Indeed, that time may be now. I highly recommend seeking out counseling or therapy as a sounding board to help you move through the complex emotions that are in your way. In the Additional Resources section of this book, I list some of the tools that have been most helpful to me on my journey.

Keep going! There's a growing bright light on the horizon.

SECTION 2

○○○— — —○○○

ACCOUNTABILITY

CHAPTER 7

Own Your Power

In my thirties, I was married with two children and living in an expensive city. I was in grad school and also our family's sole source of income. My productivity and hustle marked every day. I was fortunate to have meaningful work, but we were living paycheck to paycheck. I had to be strong and confident, yet it felt like I was holding everything together with tape, a.k.a. my force of will. In the back of my mind, I had the steady worry that everything could all fall apart in just a day, a week, or a month. This left me convinced that it should be enough to just hold onto what we already had without dreaming bigger. Maintaining my family's basic needs was the start and end of my goals.

The hard part of living this way is that there is no finish line, and it seemed like there was no time during this marathon to stop and rest or open my eyes to see what was happening around me. There was always another bill due. I dreamed of feeling better, but for the life of me, I couldn't see how to get there.

Living in California, I was surrounded, it seemed, by people who were incredibly financially well off at a young age. Their lives seemed easy, and I felt ashamed and envious that I was not experiencing the same abundance. Comparing myself to others further fed that drip, drip, drip of resentment. Perhaps, like me, you gravitate toward stories of wild successes and understandably want your own version of them. However, when we place our faith in fantasies of unexpected riches or winning the lottery, we neglect all the true prosperity and power we already possess.

Lazy Martyrdom

I spent many years hoping for things I did not have the drive or discipline to achieve, and my excuse was that everyone else's needs mattered more. In my twenties, I told myself that I would be a failure if I were not a successful writer by the time I was thirty. (I am in my fifties now, and this is the first writing project I've seen through to its intended end!) In my thirties, I was sure I needed to strike it big in the tech sector, even though I wasn't inspired to become an engineer ready to bring the next unicorn start-up to life.

After those years of unfulfilled dreams, I arrived in my forties adrift. My kids were growing up and becoming more independent, my marriage to their mother was unraveling, and I had no actionable plan, no concrete goals. I had invested so much effort in doing whatever deadening tasks needed to be done to keep my family afloat that my inner resources were utterly depleted.

The anchors of my identity as a doer were shifting, and I found myself at sea. What's crazy is that I still held on to the notion that the world would deliver what I wanted. Decades of evidence, to the contrary, had little effect on my desire to be rescued by magical forces.

Reluctantly, I began to acknowledge that my dreams would not be fulfilled simply because I was a hard-working, middle-class white man. I succumbed to depression, and my drinking entered the professional phase of its arc. What I had going on was not just passivity and fear. I had added levels of self-pity and resentment—the perfect recipe for personal toxicity.

The missing ingredient that might have countered these feelings was a sense of my power or personal agency. This is not the power that comes from wealth or status or from reacting to external requests and getting those things done. I am talking about the power that comes from knowing yourself and truly believing that your unique journey is worth showering with your attention and action. The external magical forces I was missing were actually within me. By taking myself through the process laid out in this book, I could finally see the things that would allow me to navigate life's circumstances without feeling like a victim. Instead of continuing to live as if the universe were out to get me, I felt empowered to take ownership of my happiness and personal freedom.

What's Mine?

We are sponges. Every day, all day, we soak up what is happening around us and try to make sense of it. We constantly learn and adapt, and part of that process includes absorbing the strategies and worldviews others have displayed around us.

We do this, on a most basic level, to survive. Consider what it is like to be a child: We are entirely dependent on others for all our needs, and it is in our deep interests to be lovable or do our best to fit in. And how can we best accomplish either goal? By imitating those around us.

It's often no different in our adult lives. If there is a turbulent time at work and the whole situation seems shaky, wouldn't your instinct at that moment be not to rock the boat? To fit in and not cause any trouble that might shine a spotlight on you? To do otherwise might cast you in a negative light and potentially jeopardize your access to the financial resources you need to fulfill your responsibilities.

In this context, fitting in and taking on the patterns and qualities of others is understandable. But an important part of being a mature adult is to avoid responding to situations in automatic ways. Unfortunately, when we are unconsciously parroting what we have observed in others, responding in automatic ways is precisely what we are doing.

> **An important part of being a mature adult is to avoid responding to situations in automatic ways.**

We have many ideas about ourselves, many of which have been with us for a long time. During times of stress, emotions from earlier hard times can arise that tell us that we deserve neither happiness nor success. Or they might try to convince us that nothing will be different no matter how hard we try, so we shouldn't bother. These are limiting beliefs. It does not matter if they are large or small, loud or soft; they can dominate our internal conversation and have their way with us.

Determining which limiting beliefs are *not* mine, which I've adopted from outside of myself, has opened up all sorts of space for my uniqueness to emerge. And, like many of the other processes in this book, we can begin with a single step.

For example, I have long believed *my life would be hard and overwhelming*. I have treated this as a fact. And sometimes it is, for sure, but I know I've been carrying this belief for much longer than I've been responsible for my own well-being.

If I sit with this feeling for a moment and follow it back to the earliest moment I can remember, I realize it has always been there. With this awareness, I understand that it was not something I learned through my own experience but something I took in as a very young child.

This perspective on life was not inborn for me, but it became my burden nonetheless. Just knowing that we are not the only ones responsible for the shapes of our beliefs can help take some of the pressure or negativity of such thoughts off our shoulders.

To create a bit more space between ourselves and a limiting belief, it can help to understand further what's going on by asking ourselves, "Well, if this belief is not mine, then whose is it?"

In my case, the answer was not so elusive. In the earliest years of my life, this is what was happening:

1. My father was drafted into the army during the Vietnam War and was in officer training when I was born. They gave him two days off to be at my birth.
2. After this, my parents—with both a newborn baby (me) and my eight-year-old brother—were sent to Germany for two years.
3. For a while, we shared a home with a widow and her daughter (born a day before me at the army hospital) after their husband/father was killed in combat.

4. In addition, my father had to serve his own tour of duty in Vietnam.
5. Upon returning to the states, my family settled in Palo Alto to begin a new chapter. My father wanted to finish college, and they could now accomplish other foundational goals that were ready to be taken off hold finally.
6. We found ourselves back in Arkansas, though, as circumstances evolved with the illness and passing of both my mother's parents, leaving my parents responsible for taking care of my mother's two younger sisters, who were teenagers at the time.
7. All this happened while my parents were still young, just exiting their twenties.

Okay, so that's a logical setup in which to have absorbed the lesson that life is hard and overwhelming, right? As a child, it's not even that those words occurred to me. I was soaking in the emotion and struggle that was all around me. And that's what we do as young children.

Additionally, I tried not to cause additional problems and to act as a "good boy" would. This mainly manifested in being quiet, staying out of the way, and not drawing attention to myself. This is where the classic people-pleasing strategy developed in me, a system that seamlessly followed me into adulthood. It informed the career path I chose (generally out of sight, helping to run things behind the scenes) and how I engaged in my relationships (deferring to the needs of others to avoid ruffling feathers or creating disharmony).

And now here we are, all grown up, and these younger parts are still operating inside of us, holding on to the burdens, still carrying around the internal beliefs we learned before we even had any experience of our own.

> **We can relieve our younger parts of the burdens they carry that were never theirs to hold.**

The good news is that we now have experience and skills to draw upon to rewrite these stories into something new. We can relieve our younger parts of the burdens they carry that were never theirs to hold.

Self-Reflection

Here's an exercise to address a limiting belief, access the feelings around it, and help it to shift so that its message isn't controlling your perspective any longer:

- What limiting belief have you been carrying for a long time? What's a deep-seated perspective you have that may be holding you back? The thought might begin with "I'm not . . ." or "I can't . . ." or, as with me, "Life is . . . ."
- Is there a physical feeling that arises in you as you think about it?
- Where in your body do you notice it? You may have to close your eyes to experience what part of your body is calling your attention. Take your time here to see what arises. Because we may have been bottled up for so long, distinct sensations can take a bit to separate themselves from generalized stress or tension.

- Do your best to be with the physical sensation for a moment. Is there an emotion that arises with this bodily feeling? As with the physical aspect of limiting beliefs, concise emotions can take time to gel. Stay with the process by sitting quietly, breathing steadily, and showing yourself a little patience. If nothing comes, don't worry. At the least, you have given yourself quiet space and demonstrated a genuine interest in yourself. Trying this again in a day or two may go more smoothly after a practice run.
- When an emotion makes itself known, ask yourself where it came from and when was the first time you felt it.
- Did anyone in your life at that time also seem to have this limiting belief, as evidenced by their actions or their communication with you directly?

At this point, you have done a great job listening to yourself and identifying where you learned this belief. Now it is time to engage with it. If you experience resistance or discomfort during this practice, please stop and find a less intense belief to engage with. And if you experience intense emotion, that is a good sign that you will benefit from guided professional support. (Check out the Additional Resources section at the end of the book for some places to start. If you've never had consistent professional support, commit to three visits and see how it goes. A lot can be accomplished even in that amount of time.)

So now you are engaging with a limiting belief (a burden that you carry, so to speak) that came to you from outside of your own direct experience. It is a belief or burden that you likely absorbed subconsciously for a good reason.

In my case, when I internalized the belief that life is hard, the dominating emotion I experienced was overwhelm, so naturally, I avoided engaging in situations as much as possible. Over time, I settled into a rut of avoidance, which became my comfort zone because it promised safety, if only to my young, underdeveloped self.

Self-Reflection

So, in this next exercise, please try to understand the logic behind this limiting belief. Start by asking, "What are you doing for me?" and see if any awareness surfaces. You may receive a detailed answer in response that provides some external justification, but if we look a little deeper, we will often see that the core reason for these limiting beliefs is to keep us safe.

- Thank the part of you that formed this belief for doing so much to protect you. It has worked tirelessly for years to wall you off from danger. For me, believing that life was overwhelming meant that I was less likely to stick my neck out and more likely to stay in the background.
- Let it know that you, as your skilled adult self, are now present in your life and that it would be

a shame not to engage all your skills to make a meaningful life for yourself.

- Tell the part that you are not rejecting it or banishing it. You have respect for it and want it to know that it does not have to work so hard on your behalf anymore. It can rest.
- Ask the part if you, as the present adult, can try something new. To see what is possible. And if what you try doesn't succeed, your system can see that it was not the end of the world anyway and that trying new things will not crush either of you. You can address the general sense of overwhelm by imagining a relaxing counter-moment, where you let that protective part relax and try something new. Visualize that younger part playing on the beach instead of managing your responses. Remember, one small step at a time is all that is being asked of you. With each success, our brains can relax a little, and the next step becomes more available.
- After accomplishing that simple goal, revisit the limiting belief and point out to that younger part of you that created it that you avoided feeling whatever emotion it was protecting you from and everything is okay. Pretty good.
- And since that went well, ask if you can go ahead and try another thing. Pretty soon, that part that holds the limiting belief is relaxing as well, and you are rewiring your limiting beliefs with simple, tangible steps. In other words, your experience becomes your own.

Regulate Your Reactions

Another way we can rewire our automatic responses is by working with our nervous systems. You have likely heard about being in the state of a fight, flight, or freeze response. These fight, flight, and freeze states are the extremes of our range of reactions—our most basic, core survival responses. Outside of survival situations, however, the best state to be in is generally one of calm and rational responsiveness, not fear-based or automatic reactivity to external situations. The ability to move between stressors calmly and rationally defines a regulated nervous system. There is a lot to be said about regulating the nervous system (visit Additional Resources for a little more), but touching upon it here is vital because of how it can help ease your experience of this emotional journey and any changes that present themselves.

Being in a fight, flight, or freeze mode is uncomfortable. Each of these extreme states is one of our body's natural ways of trying to protect us from physical harm. However, these states are also easily triggered by thoughts and stressful interpersonal interactions. Looking back, I can see how I likely was in a freeze state for most of my life. My general feeling of overwhelm locked me into the freeze response, which led to numbness and disconnection.

Those feelings of helplessness and overwhelm contributed even more to my general sense of powerlessness. When I quit drinking, all those unpleasant feelings were immediately more present. My nervous system needed some support if I was to become empowered in my own life and less likely to fall back into my old, unhealthy ways.

Exercise, time in nature, physical and emotional intimacy with a trusted partner, and meditation are all great ways to help ease stress and calm your nervous system. These are just some of the ingredients that keep my life balanced and happy.

Self-Reflection

In the spirit of simplicity, let's take a few minutes to discover ways to calm yourself when you feel stress coming on. Try the following suggestions to see what resonates with you the most. Pay attention to any sense of relaxation that might come on. This could be a physical release of tension, subtle tingling, deep yawn, or even a burp or fart. They can all be signs of things shifting.

If you notice any of these signs when you try out the different exercises here, that means you have found a way to support your physical self as it self-regulates while dealing with a challenging situation or emotion. As a result, you will be less likely to fall back on an unhealthy stress response like negative thinking, anger, self-pity, or helplessness or to engage in harmful and unhelpful strategies (such as all the various ways numbing yourself can show up in your life).

- Get a couple of small rubber balls, such as racquetballs, take off your shoes, sit in a chair with your low back supported, and roll your feet over them one at a time. Is there a particular part of your foot on which the pressure feels best? Next, place your feet on the balls and repeat the rolling motion. Can you feel any stress relief?

Did you notice that you were perhaps breathing a little deeper?

- Sit in a chair with your low back supported by a pillow and with both feet on the floor. Wrap your arms around your shoulders so that you are hugging yourself. Hold this posture for several minutes and observe how you unwind. Does it help to squeeze or rub your shoulders?
- Lie on your back and stretch your arms above your head to expand the distance between your fingers and your toes, taking in a deep breath. Feel into the entire length of your body. Then as you begin to slowly exhale, gently return your arms to your sides, relaxing tension out of your body. Notice what you feel and repeat 2-3 times if desired.

While seated with your back supported, breathe in for six seconds, pause for two seconds, and then exhale as slowly as possible, reaching your arms into the air as high as you can into the shape of a V, often called "victory pose."

At Home in the World

Short of retreating to the wilderness, it's impossible not to be influenced by other people. We are living in this system along with everyone else. This intertwining of our lives enables many amazing things, like our extended families, our communities, and all the ways people come together to take action and create change. This dynamic leaves us with a challenge, though: to know that we are in charge of our own happiness and fulfillment and while also needing to successfully navigate whatever people-caused challenges we may be swept up in.

We can both operate in this system and own our power, but we must be clear that our power is more than the force we use to exert our influence in the world. Nor is it something that is given to us. It is the knowledge that, simply because we exist, we are worthy of creating something unique, and when we see that we have the power to shift and change our lives, great things will happen for us *and* the world.

Unarguably, we are woven together as a people. We need each other. But we need to stop letting our well-being hinge on the reactions and actions of others. With awareness and emotional maturity, relationships can be a great source of support and happiness. But we will suffer if we give others too much responsibility for our happiness.

When we give our power to other people or situations, that lack of boundaries may make us feel taken advantage of or resentful. Hoping that others will respond to things in ways that will make us happy is a recipe for failure.

Self-Reflection

Here's an exercise to help you further unpack the ways that you engage with others:

- Consider some situations that currently upset you, either at work or home—zero in on the one that holds the most significant charge for you right now.

- Do you find that you focus on the ways other people have caused this situation?
- If you do, let everyone else off the hook for a minute. How did *you* help to set this situation in motion?
- Did you sit back and just accept how things unfolded instead of speaking up about how you feel?
- Did inaction on your part (a.k.a. passivity) fuel your resentment at the behaviors of others?
- Did your patterns and survival strategies step in to protect you and possibly make this situation more challenging than it had to be?
- Was there actual conflict attached to this situation? How would you approach it differently if you could give yourself a do-over?
- After answering these questions, do you see any themes? For example, do you tend to hang back in work meetings, so you are not called upon? Do you refrain from contributing your voice and opinions? Do you defer to your family's needs in the hope that things will be easier by doing so? Or maybe you try to communicate but get angry because you feel misunderstood?

Locating a thematic throughline of your own role in your current challenges is not easy. But once you have gained a sense of your habitual behaviors, you gain the power to revolutionize how you approach your circumstances and move through them.

CHAPTER 8

○○○— — —○○○

Face Your Fears

After so much time and energy spent deferring to others, thinking that this life of *busyness* was all that was available to me caused me a lot of pain and anxiety. This feeling of overwhelm was at the root of my passivity, and post-divorce, I faced a clear crossroads: I could continue the way I always had, which would feel safer but lead to no real happiness. Or I could make significant, potentially stressful changes to discover and fulfill my needs—which would require me to confront my fears and alter my deep-set limiting beliefs about how hard life is.

How could I create a solid plan to expand my perspective beyond the chaos happening right in front of me? As I tried to figure out where to start, I knew in my heart that I needed to deal with a pressing problem in the present moment before I could begin to plan for the future.

The behavior that stuck out to me was painfully obvious: the drinking. For so long, I had leaned on it. It held me in place, keeping me down enough that the day-to-day was all I could accomplish. It was also a problem that I could immediately address. It was a chance to take decisive action.

The Big Con

We've been told our entire lives that alcohol can be a great stress reliever, and most of us use it to deal with tension, when we socialize or to suppress uncomfortable memories and feelings we carry from our trauma. Not to mention that hanging out in bars means we surround ourselves with other drinkers, which further normalizes this behavior. Alcohol is deeply woven into our culture; for many of us, that may not be a problem. But for me, drinking had quietly and steadily grown into a significant crutch, a prop I used to handle so much of how I moved through the world.

I yearned to be happy, but I found it hard to give up doing things that I thought were helping me avoid more unhappiness. My drinking was such an obvious thing that I could change, but when it came down to it, I was afraid to commit to quitting.

Clarity came to me one day when I realized that underpinning my inability to move forward was a simple fact: I did not think I *deserved* to be happy.

It started one July morning with me at my kitchen table, asking myself again what I wanted in this life. As usual, I struggled to come up with anything specific. Usually, I would have blamed circumstances with "I'm too busy with everything in front of me to know what I want," but that day, my self-pity took the internal dialogue a little further into helplessness. A familiar part chimed in with a depressing question: "What does it really matter what I want?" In response, I felt a heaviness in my chest, like a literal brick with just one purpose: to hold me down. This negativity felt appropriate to my lack of self-worth.

I let myself feel the implications of that statement: I was *nothing* more than the roles I played. This blanket assessment of who I was in this world was hard to acknowledge, but I sat with these painful sensations and resisted the urge to push them away. There was a pointlessness and hopelessness in that viewpoint, yet I knew that it could not be the absolute truth. Where does the belief that I'm only what I do in the world make room for the love I felt for my children? There was something irreconcilable in this negativity that made me wonder if it was my truth. I could see the flaw in this viewpoint. A few minutes later, I found myself in a new place where I wanted to examine my negative attitudes with open awareness and questioning.

That was when I felt an opportunity to take an active role in caring about myself. I needed to find the strength to know that I mattered and to summon the determination to act upon that understanding. This could not be another mental exercise where I lay alone at home, asking myself a million deep questions that only led to more questions, and staring at the slowly moving ceiling fan before falling asleep. I actually had to do something.

The day before that fateful July morning, I had been actively stoking my resentments in a growler of beer, a pattern that had come to dominate my experience. That next day, to take a first step in actively caring about myself, I tackled the most obvious demon in the room. I decided to quit drinking alcohol. This sudden reversal was scary, but more than that, it was engaging. I was curious to know what could happen.

My new openness to questioning my habits and facing my fears helped to clear my mind—as did waking up without a hangover!

This lucidity helped me identify more small steps I could take to heal and feel deeply glad I was alive. My moods and outlook improved, and I saw that my anxieties (like the ones I'd held about quitting drinking) were just blinders keeping me in what I thought was my safe zone.

> **I just needed to show myself that I cared.**

This curiosity began to gain momentum within me. I was amazed that I felt pretty damn good coming out of my haze. I felt a happiness that I can only describe as an acknowledgment that I could get out of my own way. After so many years of quiet struggle, denial, self-neglect, and resentment, it was humbling to discover how accessible change was. I just needed to show myself that I cared—I had to be willing to take some basic steps to prove it to myself, which continued the momentum.

Overturning Expectations

For my entire adult life, I had stayed in the back of whatever room I was in. I'd never gotten over my seventh-grade nightmare of attempting that book report and freezing in front of the class. I wanted nothing to do with speaking in public. Yet not facing my fear of being seen or judged by others could also mean I would not step up to take the lead in situations or, ultimately, in my life.

So, when my then-girlfriend (now wife) enrolled in a three-day public speaking workshop and asked if I would join her for that weekend, I hesitated. She was nervous and thought it would be more fun to do it together. Even though I had told her repeatedly that I would do anything with her, my initial thought was, *Hell no!*

Because I had increased my ability to catch myself when reacting automatically, I recognized that this fear was possibly just some old story I was holding onto. After all, how could I know what it would be like when I had not stood in front of a group that way since childhood? And so, I acknowledged that earlier part of me who went through the bad experience in front of the classroom, who was trying to protect me from going through it again. That made a lot of sense to me; indeed, I did not want to feel that embarrassment from all those years ago. Good thing I had expanded my ability to be in the world to know that feelings wouldn't kill me!

I told my younger self that it may be scary but that no harm could come from trying. I asked myself if I might test this fear to see if it was valid. Because I was able to acknowledge the fear and not try to hide from it, emotionally, I felt more grounded, and I permitted myself to go for it. Just making that decision felt empowering, and it was a good example of putting the previously discussed parts work to use.

At the weekend workshop, I discovered that speaking extemporaneously on a topic was an exercise that part of me liked, and the environment felt safe because I knew I was in the same boat as the other students. As the weekend progressed, I watched as others went on stage before me. Everyone in the audience was happy to be there and to listen without showing any judgment. It was a space where I thought I could do things that were not typical of me.

Once that bit of comfort became available, I decided to take the speech I'd prepared a little over the top by flinging myself to the ground to emphasize a point I was making. I wanted to see if I could feel embarrassed and still enjoy myself. The old me would have thought the world would end if I made a fool of myself, but the new me made space to be surprised by what could happen.

Having a low-stakes opportunity to get on stage turned out to be fun. My classmates laughed, and I may have even helped some other nervous classmates feel permission to take the process less seriously. My experience was the exact opposite of what I thought it would be, and without a doubt, there is a direct connection between my choice to take on that new challenge and my feeling secure enough to write the book you are holding in your hands. These days, I seek what is new, unexpected, and perhaps frightening. These kind of healthy thrills continue to help me rewrite my story for myself.

> **Worries about benign and unevaluated risks are begging to be questioned and pushed back against.**

Our fears are there to protect us, but many of them operate without tangible connection to our daily reality. When fear tells me not to do a thing that holds no actual danger, something that could expand my experience, I know that it's just closing me off from my potential rather than keeping me safe. Worries about benign and unevaluated risks are begging to be questioned and pushed back against.

Self-Reflection

Confronting this aspect of your emotional life may feel like the hardest part of your journey. Believe me, though: it liberates the energy that will carry you into a life worthy of you. You have all you need to blast yourself free from the fear that constricts you, and here are some prompts to help you get there.

- First, come up with a handful of things you might dare to do if fear were not holding you back. Maybe that's camping alone, training for a marathon, skydiving, or singing or dancing in public. You know what intrigues but frightens you. That's your list.
- Next, choose the first thing on your list that leaps out at you. Jot down the thoughts, fears, and beliefs that keep you from pursuing this dream.
- Keep it light. Do not make this a deep, scary soul search, but look for limiting behaviors and beliefs that keep you from going after this desire.
- Can you think of three actions that could lessen the power of your fear over you? For example, to challenge my fear of speaking in public, I took that course, posted about it online, and found other chances to stand up and use my voice—however briefly—in front of other people. What might you do to push against your fears?
- How do you imagine your life might be different if you released this fear?
- Digest this exploration, let it sink in, select another activity from the list, and apply the same questions/prompts when ready.
- Keep in mind that pursuing what scares you can be fun. The goal is to shake things up and bring newness to your preconceived notions. What fear is holding you back that you would like to release?

When we challenge the fears holding us back, we see how we are more powerful than our worn-out strategies and that finding new perspectives is worth more than maintaining the status quo.

CHAPTER 9

Open Up to Connection

As humans, we want and need to feel connected to others to feel cared for and offer love and support. To have healthy relationships with others, we must show up for ourselves first and foremost. The more connected we are to ourselves, the easier it is for us to connect to others. Once we begin to understand and know ourselves better, we can start to take part in our relationships as our true selves. After all, don't the people in your life deserve to know the real you? Don't you deserve the opportunity to be loved for who you truly are versus just the roles you play?

> **The more connected we are to ourselves, the easier it is for us to connect to others.**

We don't need to have resolved all of our issues to engage our lives in new ways. Presenting yourself as a work in progress will be enough for people to know that you're doing your best, and their encouragement will feel good. You may be surprised at how ready some people in your life are for you to remove your self-limitations. They may well be moved by the sound of your voice catching as you express a personal truth you've kept hidden. And, as you dismantle the unhealthy coping strategies and emerge as your fuller self, your true friends and loved ones might just become your partners in shaping the life you want.

Doing things just to please others or make situations seem easier does everyone a disservice. Case in point: my people-pleasing increased the distance between me and others because I only presented myself as the person I thought they wanted me to be. Such behavior robs us of intimacy with those we love. Likewise, if we reflexively solve everyone's problems when our caretaking parts are running the show, we remove opportunities for people around us to step into their power. This is reason enough to examine our actions. Our people-pleasing habits take on a whole new significance when we consider whether we are ultimately trying to prove to other people how much they need us so that we can accommodate our insecurities. Connection to ourselves and others can only occur when we stop projecting our issues onto others and go around basing our actions on what we think others think.

Distractions Are Deadening

Suppose we think of having a good time as getting buzzed, overeating, exercising to the point of collapse, living online, or otherwise anesthetizing ourselves. Aren't we revealing that we're more content when we aren't inhabiting our lives? Yes, we can feel a lessening of daily stress when we settle in to binge-watch a new TV series or open a bottle of wine, for example, but there's a line there that's easy to cross and hard to see. If you are like me, a little numbing out quickly leads to something more serious.

The same idea applies to our phones and social media. We hop on to find something to entertain us and soften the edges of whatever we're feeling at the time (boredom, frustration, rejection, anger, etc.). As with any pleasure, our devices and virtual experiences can give us an essential boost when used in moderation. But there's that line I just described. In the same way alcohol and drugs lessen our emotional highs and lows, overindulgence in online diversions fills our time with nothingness.

Self-Reflection

Let's take a personal inventory of how, when, and why you might choose to check out:

- What are some ways that you distract yourself? (Examples are all around us, including phones, gaming, porn, overworking, drinking, and on and on.)
- When do you reach for these distractions? Are you more likely to do so at certain times of the day? What are you feeling or needing when you seek them out?
- Is there a lasting benefit to these distractions, or is the experience over when you disengage from them?
- What do you think happens to the underlying emotion(s) that led you to seek out the distraction? Does it go away? Does it still exist in you? How/where do you feel it in your body?
- How might your day be different if you sought to resolve your reason for distracting yourself directly?

Though you might argue that distractions are just there to help us pass the time, the fact is that they separate us from our emotions and personal experiences. I am not saying you must be an absolutist about staying off your phone or abstaining from any other diversion. But we need to pay attention to our behavior when we are in a place of reactivity or numbing. Central to connecting with ourselves is releasing our attachment to anything that encourages us to ignore our feelings and needs. How we feel *matters*, and this simple observation leads us to know that *we* matter. When we draw away from the emotional truth of our inner lives, we tell ourselves that we don't.

Exploring Peace Within

Connecting with ourselves is difficult when our lives revolve around external demands. There seems to be too much happening to figure out how to fit one more thing into the day. So, thinking that something needs to change is often as far as we get.

But we only need the slightest of openings to insert new perspectives into our day. With minimal effort, we can shift our ways of seeing to feel good about ourselves and make decisions that genuinely prioritize ourselves.

In moments of distress, a primary goal should be to calm our thinking minds and relax into knowing that everything is going to work out. This approach will allow us to slow down and respond to events with immediacy and genuineness. It is within our power to create a peaceful feeling that's accessible anytime, to release stress, and make our bodies comfortable places to be.

Self-Reflection

Read the imagined scene below once, going straight through. Then come back to the beginning for a slower reading. Pause a beat after each line to allow the visualization to sharpen.

Imagine yourself on an empty beach

Relaxing in the sand with your back against a warm boulder

You are younger than you are now and perhaps feel a little freer

No one needs anything from you at this moment

You can sit here without having any reason to get up

There is no one else around

Time shifts down a gear, and you become more aware of how things feel

A slight wind blows in from across the water

The sun is warm and relaxing

You hear birds squawking and look up to see them hovering in the air

They feel the sun and the wind just like you

You settle a little more deeply into the sand

You gaze over the water to the horizon

You *have the space just* to *let your curiosity wander*

And you feel yourself naturally connecting to what's around you

Sharing space with it all

You can feel a hum in your chest when you say: Here I am.

And the air around you says back: There you are.

Did you feel relaxed as you imagined the scene? Did you feel warmth circulating through you or tension releasing in your chest? If reading through the above passage was hard, can you draw a different scene in your mind that would give you a peaceful, content feeling?

If you felt a sense of serenity in your core, keep the sensation going for a little longer. Please get to know this sensation and what it feels like, so you can return to it in other settings. The aim is to develop muscle memory to let you more easily reach a place of inner calm. The next time you're waiting at an appointment, picture the beach or any setting you've replaced it with and breathe in that feeling again.

You can develop a direct channel between this connection to your inner peace and whatever you do in your day. If you're getting your tires changed and sitting in the waiting room, notice the sun shining through the window. Let it warm you, and then connect that to the more expansive experience of sinking into your surroundings. Notice the other people coming and going. Everyone has their own experience, and all we need to do now is relax into ours. There's always space to settle yourself and notice the little details that make a scene interesting and enjoyable. Pay attention. The deeper part of you wants to be curious about this life and show up for yourself. Rewrite the story that tells you to escape.

Speaking Up

The people in your life can often see your qualities (good or bad) much more clearly than you can. Knowing how hard we tend to be on ourselves, I encourage you to be open to what your loved ones communicate. If something is helpful in what they say or a truth that is hard to face, try to find gratitude. We are learning not to flee but to stay centered. Remember, you do not have to accept what others say as fact; a tough conversation can be worth it, even if the only thing that comes out of it is that you keep your calm. Well done!

The people around you are used to you being a certain way. They have long responded to how you present yourself in the world, and you have further shaped your responses based on them. Much refinement, positive and negative, goes into our strategies over time. Fortunately, we can help heal and liberate our protective parts, which have been running the show and inadvertently causing damage in our lives, with the same deliberation and steady momentum that caused them to take on their roles in the first place.

> **We are learning not to flee but to stay centered.**

Your desire to change needs to be clear to the people around you because once you begin to do things differently, they will likely adapt their behavior. In the past, my view of relationships was rooted in the notion that we all must compete to meet our individual needs. And wanting to avoid conflict, I employed passive-aggressive (or even destructive) tactics to try and get the upper hand. To get out of this cycle, I had to step up and speak my needs—to make changes in my behavior and not be afraid to do so. Even if our requests aren't met immediately, we are exercising our ability to communicate on our behalf, and this capacity grows through successes and failures alike. We all win if the people we care about are receptive to our needs. If they aren't receptive to our needs or discourage our growth, we have learned important information about the true nature of these relationships and can reassess how/if they fit into our life.

Allow yourself the freedom to make the first steps toward unlocking who you are without trying to gameplan for how others will respond. Just be brave, do it, and know that the outcome will certainly not be as bad as you imagine.

Suppose you are in a pattern of keeping your feelings under wraps. In that case, you will be surprised by how much improving your communication and releasing many of the desires and emotions you hold bottled up within yourself will lead to positive change.

When we've deferred to the needs of others for so long, we need to find a simple starting point in voicing our needs and wants in positive and productive ways. If we were to jump straight into the deep end of the communication pool with this project, we would likely create more conflict than resolution. That's because we are still learning to connect to ourselves and convey our concerns, independent of what goes on around us. These are skills that we have to build actively.

Self-Reflection

For the first practice listed here, find a friend with whom you have a reasonably simple, low-stress relationship. You don't need anything from one another other than to set aside half an hour to chat. Be sure to choose someone who can keep this experience to themselves so that you're not wondering how it would sound to anyone else. This person will sit across from you and listen, neither reacting nor giving advice.

Here's what I want you to do. In front of your friend, respond to the following prompts aloud:

- List a few goals that would cause you to be excited about your future. Don't think small. Dream big.
- Do you feel more excited about one of these? Why is that? Does it align with what's expected of you, or does it represent something in you that wants to be expressed? Explain that this goal is rising to the top of what you want to get done.
- How does it feel to express this dream out loud? Maybe you feel inspired? Some nervousness? Perhaps a bit of clarity!
- Are there any initial steps you could take to move down the path to making this happen?

- Can you connect to this dream enough to look at your friend and say, "This is important to me—I want this to happen"?

The friend is simply there to witness you as you voice your dreams. If the opportunity interests them, they can weigh in to support you with ideas for the next steps. You can reverse the roles and listen to them share if they would like to.

Self-Reflection

The next step is to expand on what you learned from this conversation and engage with your partner or someone close to you with whom your life is intertwined and with whom there may be a misunderstanding or competing needs.

Keep in mind that this next version of the exercise will require a level of patience that was not needed when you were talking with your friend. You will now share what you have discovered with someone who is used to you behaving a certain way or being predictably reliable. Because you may have competing interests around specific topics, this exercise will encourage you to stay in your experience (remember the grounding exercise if you feel your heart rate ticking up, your breath quickening, or your body tensing) while also communicating your needs. Mixing and matching healthy communication and grounding skills will accelerate the growth you seek.

To get a conversation off on the right foot, it can be helpful to put up some guard rails with the other person so that you both know what to expect and when to take a break. We all know how quickly supposedly simple conversations can go sideways. We must create space in our relationships to be honest about what we want and who we are.

Our partner (or whomever we are going deep with) will also benefit from feeling safer in the conversation. With practice, we can get good at introducing thoughts, feelings, or ideas to another person without anyone getting defensive. And conversation can be an excellent way to welcome creativity into our relationships.

To that end, here are a few ground rules to keep in mind. Add to them as you wish.

- Be patient with yourself and others. This is new territory.
- Speak when it's your time to speak, and listen when it's time to listen.
- Don't assign blame. It takes two to be in a relationship, so we share responsibility for situations.

Here's how you might introduce a topic:

YOU: "I'm reading a book that suggests learning to be more open about what's going on in my life. I hope this will ultimately make things easier for me and us.

> Can we try an exercise together? We can each try out both sides of the conversation if you want. That way, I'm working on listening too."
>
> *Or*
>
> YOU: "I want to learn to talk more about what's going on with me. It's not that I want to talk about any issues, really. It's just that I don't even know how to bring things up before they've become problems staring me in the face."
>
> You get the idea. We want to frame the exercise as an overall improvement in how we interact with others. We want to add this to our skill set around communicating our needs.
>
> Something else you can do to take some of the heat off trying to get the language right the first time is to give each other some free passes. For example:
>
> YOU: "Because this personal communication stuff is new to me, I need to be able to make mistakes and know everything will still be okay. So, can I have three do-overs per month for anything I say that I want to take back? I'll give you free passes, too, if you want."

In a spirit of appreciation toward yourself and your commitment to living your life in new ways, try out some new ways of sharing that might feel awkward but have the potential to shorten the emotional distance between you and the person with whom you're sharing. Be patient with yourself and ask others to be patient with you too.

I don't know about you, but for me, expressing my feelings and desires out loud was terrifying for most of my life. Keeping the truth of ourselves hidden from people we care about, though, means we don't get to partake of this powerful web that links all human life. That's a loss I would consider downright tragic. I encourage you to dip your toe in the waters of deeper relationships. I suspect you will find deep relief and great joy in telling the world what's on your mind.

SECTION 3

ACTION

CHAPTER 10

Create Momentum

Connecting with myself outside my role of doer was revolutionary. The more I witnessed this long-suppressed self, the more being authentically me became non-negotiable. It started with the question of what would happen if I changed just one destructive behavior (drinking), and once I had that answer (nothing bad!), I wanted to question the next dubious story circulating in my mind. After we take our first steps toward change, the transformation can build beautifully upon itself. Making brave new choices becomes natural, and making the right personal decisions becomes a new standard.

> **After we take our first steps toward change, the transformation can build beautifully upon itself.**

Awareness Leads to Accountability

When I stopped using booze to flee my emotional life, I began thinking more clearly and seeing beyond the day-to-day. A path appeared. One act of self-care led to another and another. The ease of being myself was so tangible that I wanted more. I sought the company of other people who were asking questions of themselves.

I woke up without sluggishness or a headache and took walks or went to a meditation group. Time for myself just appeared.

I began to disentangle myself from my patterns and gained increasing perspective. I could trace a direct line from my passive inaction as a man to the fear activated in me as a child. Acting on my pledge to take risks, I committed to my work with my therapist, who knew how to take me to the beginnings of my various fears safely. I learned how to be with my emotions, acknowledge them, and finally start to let them go.

The ability to examine these feelings but not be consumed by them also allowed me to recognize how they had informed my decades of living. Empowered with this view, I could spot where and when fear would likely pop up next, and having an awareness of my nervous system meant that it was less likely to take control of me. As a skilled adult finally gaining some emotional maturity, I became increasingly able to disengage from the habitual reactions that had always led to internal chaos.

Accountability Leads to Action

I've learned that we must dig into the deep stuff to live passionately in the present. May I be so bold as to say that this is a fact? I tried for decades to avoid looking into my emotional wounds and always ended up in the same place. I kept trying to put a bandage on the present instead of looking to the past because I was overwhelmed by the pain that I imagined was waiting for me there.

Healing from childhood trauma is not an easy process. Whether or not you've experienced abuse, when we begin to unearth old wounds, at moments, the flood of emotion can feel like too much. Painful memories can pop up and demand our attention. As we assess the impacts of fear and pain on our present lives, we might feel sadness or guilt that we haven't been the parent or partner we think we should have been. Professional guidance and support are highly recommended.

But once your energy starts to get unstuck, you won't want to return to the flatness of coping and getting by. The sudden access to powerful emotions (even the painful ones) and the support and tools to move them can be a welcome wake-up call to the numbed-out system—one of those moments when we can further proclaim: "Here I am."

Action Leads to Change

Once the process got rolling, digging down and addressing my core wounding took months, not the years I'd expected. That is not to say that I am done healing or that internal struggles do not creep up anymore. But the difference between the person I was when I first took the leap to start caring about myself and the person I was six months later is like the difference between two separate people. I find this remarkable, especially when I contrast my current life with the decades I spent being depleted, reactive, frustrated, angry, and insecure. I challenge you to take your life into your hands and deal with anything buried that's keeping you stuck, and I recommend finding a trusted professional to support you (see the resources section at the back of the book). We are all entitled to the happiness and freedom that's on the other side of facing our demons.

From my own experience, here are a few new guiding truths:

- Looking in the mirror, feeling our feelings, and embracing change are much less painful options than struggling to maintain a false sense of control.
- The energy we put into living in survival mode is vastly more exhausting than the energy it takes to dig into healing and experimenting with new ways of being.
- The few things we might risk by being proactive and making changes are rarely as scary as we imagine they will be.

Slight Hiccups

Sometimes, we backslide and find ourselves mired in our old fears or patterns. This is human, and I've experienced this quite recently. While focusing on the second draft of this book, I lost my enthusiasm, which was strange because I have been excited to connect with you through my story. So, what was going on?

When I tried to renew my focus, the disconnection turned to a nervous dread in my chest, and a jumble of negative thoughts crowded my mind. The one message that rose above the others was a simple "It will be easier just to stop." This assertion landed one day with such certainty that I felt for a moment that it must be my truth. When a part of us takes over our system, it can feel like an unshakeable truth rather than a part trying to protect us at that moment.

I sat on the couch quietly for a few minutes and let my breath even out. That created some space for my curiosity to show itself. And so I asked, "Why am I so scared of finishing my book?"

And the part of me voicing fear provided a list of things that could happen:

- I am not a professional writer, and people might think my book sucks.
- I am not a teacher or a philosopher. Why should I expect to be able to share wisdom?
- My family will be embarrassed that I shared my challenges and pain.
- By making my childhood abuse public, my general feelings of shame will be magnified a million times over.
- People will think that I'm arrogant.
- No one will care.

Wow! That's quite a range. Any one of those would be a good enough excuse to call it quits should I want to. I mean, we half-ass start projects that don't go anywhere all the time, right? And besides, I got most of this book written and learned some things about how I operate. That's *good enough.*

But because of that breathing I took the time for, I let these thoughts settle. I saw how that attitude of *good enough* would keep me small. Wow again! Layer upon layer of personal resistance was at play.

I decided to address each of the fears logically. In chapter 8, we looked at the power that can come from confronting our fears. I return to that subject here more granularly to show how conversing with our fear and examining what scares us is crucial to claiming our own lives. I have found that with practice, it's possible to be present with our fears and break them down into little pieces, and those segments tend not to hold up to healthy emotional scrutiny. Because each fear was trying to protect me, I decided to respect it enough to hear it out. I asked my fear to let the part of me excited by the book respond. That felt fine, so off we went:

- FEAR: I am not a professional writer, and people will think my book sucks.

  RESPONSE: Everyone who puts something creative into the world probably feels insecure, but they do it anyway because they are called to, and taking a risk like this probably makes their lives more meaningful. Why should it be any different for me?

- FEAR: I am not a teacher nor a philosopher. Why should I expect to be able to share wisdom?

  RESPONSE: That's a fear straight from the ego. I don't need to be "wise." I just want to connect with my readers in a positive, productive way, sharing insight I believe could be useful to them.

- FEAR: My family will be embarrassed that I shared my challenges and pain.

  RESPONSE: This is a pretty good one! I can decide not to follow through because doing so would protect others. That's classic people-pleasing logic. But I believe they would rather see me being authentically me than staying trapped in resentful misery.

- FEAR: By making my abuse public, my general feelings of shame will be magnified by a million.

  RESPONSE: Another excellent excuse and one that does hold some weight. Vulnerability is hard. Ultimately, I must trust in my mission to be of support to others. I also know that by stepping into my power and owning my experience, I am rewriting my story of being a scared little boy. And I know that sharing my vulnerability can inspire others and that I'm not alone in my experience.

- FEAR: People will think that I'm arrogant.

  RESPONSE: I need to let myself off the hook on this. I can't guess how others will respond to me, especially when I am trying something they do not expect from me. If I act in good conscience and others still speak ill of me, let's consider that their thoughts about me might be their projections about themselves.

- FEAR: No one will care.

  RESPONSE: For this one, I turned to the fear and said, "You may be right, and if so, that makes for an even stronger case to finish this project since nothing negative will come of it. If nothing else, I can put my stamp on this moment and declare that I was here."

Following this conversation with myself, I turned back to that feeling of dread that was encouraging me to leave the book unfinished. Because I had hollowed out all its arguments, it was reduced to nothing but hot air. That dread that just a bit ago had me locked up suddenly lost its power. My fear saw that there was now a mature adult in the room, and it could let go of being in charge. It no longer needed to search for reasons not to be brave because it could see that I had become plenty able to respond to challenges. All the life skills we've discussed came to pay off in a new way for me.

Can you try this for yourself when you next get the chance? When fear comes knocking, can you ask it to be specific so you can present a different viewpoint? This is another way we can exercise our voice, an internal way. Being in dialogue with your difficult inner voices shows that the mature, present part of you is not rejecting your challenges. By being curious about your own life, you deepen the bond with your own experience and are less likely to let fear derail you from the path to making change.

> **When fear comes knocking, can you ask it to be specific so you can present a different viewpoint?**

It can start with something as simple as asking a question. We need to directly address our challenging emotions before we can break our patterns and invite in something new and inspiring. Find something that you would like to question. See if it holds up to loving scrutiny. I know that you can do it.

CHAPTER 11

○○○— — —○○○

Explore Your Purpose

Our personal exploration contains an inherent acknowledgment of the mystery and complexity of our lives. Now that my feet are on the ground and I've grown up a bit, I am in awe of this. Why would Nature create complex animals like us with so much mental and emotional baggage? To me, it seems that reason is to learn and evolve.

The Wildness of Life

I invite you to step outside into the daylight. In a simple moment such as this, we can quickly access a perspective on what is happening that goes well beyond our normal observations. Science tells us that though the light that warms your skin took only eight minutes to travel from the Sun to the top of your head, it took thousands of years to escape the gravity of the Sun's core, where it was born. And here *we* are, gangly creatures who go to extraordinary lengths to get in our own way. How can all of this be happening at the same time?

That this intricate and dazzling world exists and that we are here to witness it informs me that there is more to our human existence than what we see and feel. There's *something* more here. To me, this curiosity is an aspect of the soul. We strive to learn and grow through our experiences, and the lessons of this life are more significant than we may want to face. Yet we do. There's a purpose.

Nature and Nurture

Since our brains are soaking up so much external input from the moment we're born, it's no wonder our feelings and reactions come flying fast. This quick start in our nervous systems occurs as we assess every moment according to the basics: Are we safe? Are we loved? Are we nourished? We are born into this constant swirl of experience, which only ends when we pass. To stand fully as our unique selves in the chaos, we must have our feet on solid ground. The best and most fun way to do so is to feel connected to our deepest feelings and desires, and that requires acknowledging and healing from the hard stuff.

> **To stand fully as our unique selves in the chaos, we must have our feet on solid ground.**

Actively appreciating the bigger picture has kept my curiosity in high gear and given me the sense that we are never alone, no matter how isolated we might feel on a bad day. It may be the same for you. Can you make space to consider the bigger picture of what is happening in the world? Please consider these three related concepts that feel true to me as I've pondered deeper meaning in my life:

- There must be more to this strange and complex world than meets the eye.
- Nature seeks balance and logically guided progress through cause and effect. People are not always logical and can be blind to the causes and effects we experience and perpetuate.
- The harmony of Nature is not necessarily reflected in our own lives. To experience it, we need to expand outside the narrow view provided by our daily perceptions and see life with fresh eyes.

What does your curiosity tell you about life and our place in it?

Higher-Level Direction

Do you feel a sense of awe when pondering the universe and our place on this piece of rock flying through space? How amazing is it that, along with the stars and planets, there is also *you*? You, with all of your complexity, energy, and creativity. The universe has made a great effort to bring you here, which is a perfect acknowledgment of why your individual experience is worth exploring and expanding.

> **Your individual experience is worth exploring and expanding.**

Seeing ourselves in this greater context can further open us up to a perspective that contains so much more than what we see going on around us. We can walk a path that reveals opportunities specific to us and enables us to tap into our most inherent abilities. Two avenues for charting your desired course are identifying your highest values and creating a personal mission statement.

Think of your values as the things that light you up. We each have unique blends of what activates and inspires us. When we are engaged with these aspects of ourselves, the rest of our lives becomes more vibrant. There are many tools online for identifying your values; you can also find one in the Additional Resources section at the end of the book. The process does not take long, and it's fun to see what's uncovered.

Through my own exploration, I found that my highest value is a solid connection to my inner life. I naturally seek to understand my experience. However, this characteristic was not always clear to me since I spent so many years disconnected from myself. That's how it can be for us humans. The most important things for our growth and evolution often hide in our blind spots.

Writing this book has allowed me to exercise this highest value of mine. Regardless of who reads it, diving into this project has played an essential role in my self-exploration.

My second highest value is a connection to my environment. If you could see me at home right now, you'd know the intensity with which I focus on maintaining my surroundings. A complementary aspect of being a neat freak is that I also get to find inspiration and get creative in my personal space.

These two aspects of my personality shed light on my long-term dream to organize my days so that for half of my time, I'm using my brain to know myself—and using this understanding to move through the world in a way that feeds me instead of wears me out—and for the other half, I'm blissed out pulling weeds in the garden and cooking the food that I grew.

Discovering your top values can help you see your life more expansively and help guide your decisions, even allowing you to foresee and plan for future transitions. And by connecting to our different values, we can better soothe ourselves during challenging times. For example, suppose I am feeling down about something significant in my life. In that case, the experience is not so draining or overwhelming when I also have the comfort of my relaxing personal space.

Life on Purpose

Once you've determined your highest values, your life's purpose—something I refer to as a personal mission statement—flows from and serves your highest values. As with the previous section on personal values, a good resource is provided at the back of the book to assist.

Knowing what matters most to you can strengthen your sense of purpose and vice versa. Drafting a personal mission statement can be a profound act of self-discovery. And though it may evolve and change as you do, having a mission statement can function as a North Star, offering orientation when you feel lost at sea. For help creating your mission statement, check out the Additional Resources section at the end of this book.

My experience composing a mission statement has evolved as I have become better connected to myself, and the personal changes I've undergone are evident in the language of each version. Your mission statement can be updated when necessary as your connection to yourself deepens and becomes increasingly sturdy.

The first time I created one was in my early forties, as an assignment for a course I was taking. I worked hard on it and felt pride in the goals it expressed. I thought that it represented the best aspects of my place in the world:

I am change, and I am not afraid to act. I explode economic and societal boundaries and limitations through inspired action and *connection to others.*

What I realized about this statement is that this is not my personal mission—it's my ideal mission for work. It talks about what I do in collaboration with other people, not who I am at my deepest core. I can understand how I arrived at this confusion. My work life in my twenties began in the trucking industry and ended with working in industrial health and safety at a steel fabrication plant. Those jobs were exhausting experiences that paid the bills but did not interest me. On my thirtieth birthday, I moved with my family to California. I quickly moved into the nonprofit space, supporting sustainable businesses to become more socially and environmentally responsibly. What a change from my previous work experiences!

I was so deep into fulfilling my obligations via this more fulfilling work that I could not see where work ended and my personal experience began. It can be great to express a mission statement for your work that will help guide your decisions, but it should not be confused with who you are. It makes sense that the confusion I experienced is what can happen when you cannot see yourself beyond what you do in the world.

I sat with that existing mission statement for a bit, feeling around it to see what was at its core. When I incorporated the two values referenced above (inner life and environment) into a new statement, here's what I came up with:

My purpose is to fearlessly explore my inner life,
my personal story, and how I relate to the world
so that I can both create change in myself and
inspire others to do the same.

Now we're getting somewhere! I can see myself in this statement; it feels closer to something I can call my own. But, as a mission statement, it is a little clunky, and I can tell that I was still mostly approaching it with my logical, reasoning mind.

So, what is in there that gets to the very center of who I am? "Fearlessly explore" resonates, and I often need something that strong to get me to address the muck in my life and step into something bigger. Another way to express this is to say that I enjoy exploring healing. And as in the previous version, whatever I'm accomplishing, I would like to inspire others to do the same.

And then it came to me in a lean eight words:

My purpose is to fearlessly inspire others to heal.

Since it is helpful to make your mission an active statement instead of just declarative, mine then became:

I fearlessly inspire others to heal.

It is short and sweet. It gives me goosebumps when I say it. It is simultaneously audacious and giving. And it has real-life power.

It gave me the necessary accountability to finish this book when my fear said it would be easier not to.

The first time I said those six words together, I got choked up. If you feel that emotion as you find your statement, it will be a good marker that you're on to something hugely true.

> **Fulfilling your mission means that you will show up in brand new ways and be acknowledged for new reasons.**

Ideally, your mission statement should scare you a little, too. After all, fulfilling your mission means that you will show up in brand new ways and be acknowledged for new reasons. Of course, you could already be living a good portion of your mission because, deep down, you were pulled toward what holds meaning. If that's the case, then congratulations on stumbling upon it! If not, enjoy finding your purpose and committing to it with language. It's an eye-opening process and one that can bring much happiness.

CHAPTER 12

○○○— — —○○○

Ever-Expanding You

So much of the magic in our lives is made of things we didn't see coming. When we were just getting by in our static roles, we had to sell ourselves on a false sense of control. Often when we've felt unsafe in our lives, parts of us took on the role of trying to establish a sense of control. That's a big, stressful order and destined to fail. One of the ways we maintain a sense of control is by making our worlds more constricted, smaller, and manageable. We were either placing ourselves into boxes or allowing others to do it for us.

Living in our true power gives us perspective on where we've come from, engages us in the present moment, and offers us a sense of where we want to go. We become confident in our abilities and connected to our needs. This allows us to be more open to whatever may happen and embrace the possibilities that await us.

Be Your Own Best Friend

I encourage you to be patient with yourself as you gain new perspectives on your habits and feel your unhealthy patterns start to unwind. As deeply held viewpoints begin to shift and we breathe a little deeper, we can drop into trust in our new insights and awareness of the moment. The relaxing connection to ourselves is an excellent indicator that we are making progress.

The more you put guidance in this book into practice, the more natural it all becomes. Playfulness can grow out of this process because the outcomes feel so palpably good. If you've read this far, you are already connecting to yourself. You are likely approaching your life with a new force of intention. Think about the possibilities unfurling before you. Time spent pursuing personal change will be a reward in and of itself. If you haven't already, you will find that you like who you are. The accomplishments that happen because you devoted yourself to developing awareness, accountability, and action in your life become the icing on the cake.

> **Time spent pursuing personal change will be a reward in and of itself.**

Increasingly, I am amused when I see myself trying to slip back into old patterns. Because I am better rooted in the present, I can acknowledge these familiar tugs without fear and allow them to remind me of how far I've traveled. I thank them for showing me where I was before and how much more joyful I am now.

Beyond the Daily Grind

You can do lots of good things in the world before you even have a sense of purpose to guide you. However, your level of connection to your activities will be much higher when you are doing the things that make you who you are. Until I wrote the words *I inspire others to heal*, I had never challenged myself to be a public-facing person in any meaningful way. And now, because I have identified this mission for myself, I must run toward the things that will help me fulfill it. Wallflower that I once was, I now place myself in front of others, through this book and in various ways, face to face.

What do we want for ourselves? I imagine we've all got universal wants mixed in with our specific desires. From a ten-thousand-foot view, I want to love myself and continue to grow. This means I am responsible for examining my decisions and state of mind. I give myself permission to be patient with situations, improve them as I can, and step away if needed. Can you name one of your stronger desires for yourself?

Now that you are connecting more authentically with yourself, let's see what magic can happen when you take the time to establish some broad personal standards.

Here are a few declarative statements that keep me aligned with my mission and guide me in how I want to live. I believe that if I follow them, the details of my life will flow with greater ease because I am now combining my hard-earned skillset with my inspiration.

- I want to be aware of my challenges and blind spots and not be afraid or overwhelmed by them.
- I want relationships that do not involve us playing out our pain with one another.
- I want to be confident in my abilities rather than competitive with others.

- I want to be a healthy resource for those around me, especially those who need me.
- I want to be proud of the scars that have made me who I am and use them to create a fuller version of myself than I thought possible.

I can achieve these goals because I am increasingly focusing my energy on my desires and living authentically as myself.

Self-Reflection

It's time to set some goals for yourself. What declarations would you like to make about your life? There are endless possibilities that can be changed whenever a new one comes your way. Make them both substantial and achievable. Let them represent this new, expanded version of yourself.

- Choose three goals you want to accomplish in the next year and five more to complete within three to five years.
- Build out the story for each goal by describing how life will be different once you achieve it.
- In what ways will they build your connection to yourself and the world?
- What initial steps can you take to bring these goals to life?
- And do some excite you more than others? Do some seem more achievable? Give attention to any that make you tingle.

Getting Real

Our fears are tiny compared to the reality of who we are. I am reminded of this when I reflect on the rollercoaster of responsibilities I spent so long choosing to ride, instead of being brave for my own sake. The choices I eventually made to change this dynamic often felt too big and scary for me, but that's all part of the illusion.

With your newly unclouded eyes, you may see that the most significant limits on your experience are those you've placed upon yourself. Consider all you have accomplished and how strong you are even though you've spent years performing for others. Now that you've opened up to knowing yourself more fully, you are at the helm of your own life, not blaming others or outside forces for your circumstances. You're now empowered to enjoy the responsibility of creating your own unique, engaging, and beautiful life.

ADDITIONAL RESOURCES

This section will direct you to some of the tools presented in this book. Take them as food for thought, or perhaps pledge to incorporate the ones that intrigue you most into your own life. Consider these resources and positive steps you can take to create personal freedom and happiness.

1. Parts Work/Internal Family Systems (IFS) – This method of examining why we repeat unhealthy patterns was a real life-changer for me. Receiving support for your day-to-day challenges is important; however, I've found that you must go to the source of your strategies and perspectives to make the changes that keep your old daily story from repeating itself. Visit this site to find someone who might also help you: www.ifs-institute.com/practitioners. You can also begin by reading *No Bad Parts* by Dr. Richard Schwartz. He created IFS and is a very accessible writer. You can also go search online for interviews and presentations by him that explain the process in very clear ways.
2. Nervous System Support – A simple web search provides many resources for understanding and soothing your nervous system. If you want to gain a deeper understanding of this vital part of your body's operating system and learn practical

exercises to regulate your responses to life's challenges better, I recommend this resource: www.traumahealingaccelerated.com/programs/

3. Eye Movement Desensitization and Reprocessing (EMDR) – Just like our nervous system, our brain can also benefit from a little direct TLC. EMDR uses sound or vibrations (among other things) to help rewire our brain's responses when we think about challenging situations or memories. EMDR can be explored independently, but I found it most potent when used in conjunction with IFS (see above) and professionally guided support. Here's general information: www.emdr.com/what-is-emdr/

4. Values Assessment – What are the aspects of your life that light your fire? When we make decisions and behave in ways aligned with our values, life feels more meaningful and we have a greater chance for happiness. There are lots of resources for exploring your value system, and here is a great, free place to start: www.drdemartini.com/values/

5. Mission Statement – Defining your purpose as a mission statement is one of the best things you can do to elevate your experience in this life. What's your North Star? What do you see as your unique contribution to the world during this life? Let's find out! Remember that the statement can be a living thing that gets refined over time as you learn more and your experience evolves. Visit my website at www.nathanjoblin.com/bookgift and download a worksheet to help create your mission statement.

6. My Website – I am invested in your growth and evolution and want to stay connected with you on your journey. Please visit www.nathanjoblin.com for more offerings, including an online course based on the material covered in this book.

ACKNOWLEDGMENTS

First, thank you to my book coach and partner, Catherine, for the steady encouragement and accountability. Thanks also to the editorial and design team for their support and expertise: Madeleine, Dave, and Minhaj, with special thanks to Melinda and Gabi for always rising to the occasion when I needed them.

Deep appreciation goes out to my friends Matt, Chris, and Adam, who stepped up and participated as I explored how to put the contents of this book together in a logical way.

A big thank you goes to Ian Birlem for showing me how to navigate my challenging emotions and understand why I behaved the way I did. Thanks also to Reuvain Bacal for introducing new and easeful ways to communicate, both as an individual as well as in coupledom.

My gratitude goes out to all of the clients at Modern Wisdom Press. Your bravery in stepping up and writing your book inspired me to keep writing when it was most difficult. To the *Trapped* launch team members and its advance readers, thank you for helping to build awareness of this book.

My family gets a special shoutout for accompanying me in this life. I wouldn't be here without you!

ABOUT THE AUTHOR

○ ○ ○ — — — ○ ○ ○

Nathan Joblin

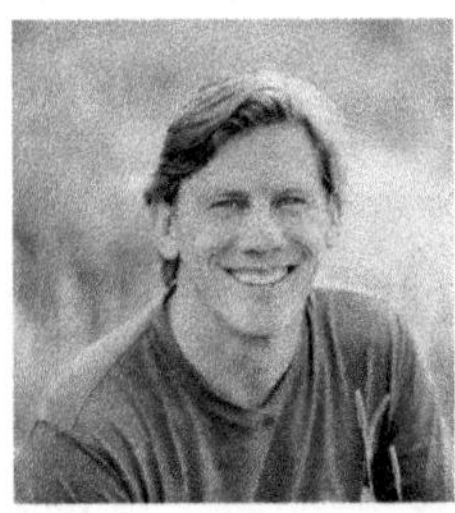

NATHAN JOBLIN is the COO + Co-Founder of Modern Wisdom Press. His journey to becoming a published book author inspires him to support clients in overcoming the obstacles to sharing their message with the world.

His passion for operations includes decades in the publishing, nonprofit, and education sectors, with various organizations supporting sustainable alternatives to business. Nathan earned his bachelor's degree from Amherst College and his master of science in Environmental Management from the University of San Francisco.

Nathan lives a full life as an entrepreneur, father, husband, and caretaker of a high-energy dog, a lazy cat, and two demanding donkeys on a few acres in Colorado. He finds pleasure in the solitude of walks in the woods and his daily meditation and breathing practices. Regardless of the number of responsibilities on his plate, Nathan is always scouting out his next opportunity for adventure, specifically where he can explore new cultures, practice his Spanish, and throw on a mask and snorkel to get lost in the mysteries of the underwater world.

THANK YOU

○○○— — —○○○

I hope this book has served you well and that you are already introducing new ways of living into your daily experience. One of my goals is to continue to provide perspective and connection and so please visit my site at www.nathanjoblin.com for information on course and event offerings.

www.ingramcontent.com/pod-product-compliance
Lightning Source LLC
Chambersburg PA
CBHW022059020426
42335CB00012B/754

9781951692322